THE VAGUS NERVE

Polyvagal Theory: Activated and access the healing power of the Vagus Nerve. Psychological and emotional manipulation with self-help exercises for trauma depression, Yoga Anatomy

Dr. Jason Mayer

TABLE OF CONTENTS

INTRODUCTION

Congratulations on purchasing *The Vagus Nerve,* and thank you for doing so.

The following chapters will discuss what the vagus nerve is, what it controls, what can happen when it is compromised, stimulation treatment, and homeopathic therapy. It will explore the connection between vagus nerve health, mental health, physical health, and resilience. Hopefully, you will walk away with tips, techniques, and the motivation to maintain or restore your vagus nerve resilience.

There are plenty of books on this subject on the market, thanks again for choosing this one! Every effort was made to ensure it is full of as much useful information as possible. Please enjoy!

CHAPTER 1

Overview

Why read a book about the vagus nerve? It would behoove everyone, especially if you live in the United States of America, to understand the implications of a healthy vagus nerve. The U.S. has become one of the least healthy, happy, or safe nations in the world.

Commonwealthfund.org published an article in May 2020 titled, Mental Health Conditions and Substance Use: Comparing U.S. Needs and Treatment Capacity with Those in Other High-Income Countries. It compared the mental health of the world's wealthiest nations. According to this article, the United States of America has the highest suicide rate in the industrialized world. Furthermore, it has the fewest resources to help those struggling.

The United States also ranks poorly in education. Thirty years ago, we ranked 6th in the world. Today we rank 27th, according to a 2018 Business Insider article. Part of that may be because of spending, but multiple sources blame it on diet, technology, and social media.

Our physical health isn't any better. According to a 2018 Forbes article, U.S. Health Outcomes Compared to Other Countries Are Misleading, the United States has the highest obesity rate. With 36.5 percent of the population classified as obese, many other comorbidities are involved. Diabetes is commonly associated with obesity and, with all its complications, is the third leading cause of death.

We aren't even a very safe or friendly nation. We have one of the worst rates of gun violence-related deaths in the world. The U.S. death rate related to guns was 10.6 per 100,000 people in 2016. This ranking is much higher compared to Canada (2.1 per 100,000) and Australia (1.0), France (2.7), Germany (0.9), and Spain (0.6).

From physicians to politicians, from pastors to police, all these professionals are treating the problems separately. But what if they are all the same problem? What if you can trace these seemingly disparate issues plus a plethora of other morbidities to one root cause? Maybe this is why you should be reading a book about the vagus nerve.

Besides all of the above, it is really quite a fascinating nerve. It is instrumental in the control and maintenance of every one of your major body systems. It is the reason you can relax at night after a hard day's work. It is why you can talk and sing. You couldn't chew and swallow your food without it, nor could you digest your food. Are you breathing? Is your heart beating? That's because of the vagus nerve. Signals carried by the vagus nerve also control your ability to heal and your immune response. Even your mental health is affected by the vagus nerve.

Structures of the Nervous System

Before we embark on a full discovery of the vagus nerve, though, a basic understanding of the nervous system, in general, would be a good foundation. You probably learned all about it in school, but here's a refresher. The nervous system is a remarkable and complex electrical network of nerve cells. Sometimes we may refer to nerve cells as neurons or nerve fibers. Your science teacher may have had you look at your hand in school and imagine that your palm was the nerve cell body, and your fingers were the dendrites reaching out to touch a target. Your teacher may have also explained using the hand metaphor, that the arm was the axon. And just as the electrical cords in your house need to be covered by a protective coating, most nerve cells also have a protective covering called the myelin sheath. So, imagine your arm is surrounded by sweatbands to complete this visual of the neuron.

Neurons send or receive information in the form of electrical impulses that travel along the entire cell's length. The dendrites pick up a signal and pass it into the cell body and on to the axon. The axons, which can be up to a few feet long in larger animals, send the signal to their target. But they don't touch the destination. Instead, there are tiny spaces called synapses between the axon and the target. A chemical called a neurotransmitter is needed to carry the electrical impulse across that space. The goal can be the dendrites of another neuron, or it can be the cells of an organ or a gland.

Cells that carry information *to* the spinal cord or brain, such as sensory neurons, are called afferent neurons. In contrast, cells carrying information *away* from the spinal cord or brain, such as motor neurons, are called efferent neurons. These will be essential terms, so let's review them now. If a neuron approaches the central nervous system, it is called afferent (<u>a</u>pproaching is <u>a</u>fferent with an <u>a</u>). If a neuron exits the central nervous system, it is called efferent (<u>e</u>xiting is <u>e</u>fferent with an <u>e</u>). Bundles of these neurons are called nerves or nerve tissue. When a nerve interacts with other cells, it is said to innervate them. The motor nerves may serve muscle cells, and sensory nerves may innervate, or serve, taste buds. The entire nervous system, made up of these nerve bundles, can be divided into two main categories. These categories include the central nervous system and the peripheral nervous system.

The Central Nervous System

The central nervous system is centrally located right in and on top of the center of our spine. Also, it is fundamental to where all the information is sent and received. It consists of the brain and the spinal cord. We won't spend much time here, although its mysteries and complexities fill volumes of books on the subject. We'll just concentrate on the main structures right now. Our brain consists of three main parts; the cerebrum, the cerebellum, and the brain stem. These sections work together to relay information back and forth to keep everything functioning in perfect harmony.

The cerebrum is the most extensive section of the brain. It is the noodle-looking gray matter with two hemispheres and is what we typically think of when we recall an image of the brain. The cerebrum is where we think and reason, process sensory information and coordinate our movements. You're using your cerebrum right now to read this and recall pictures of brains you've seen in the past. It has two nerve pairs that directly connect to it, which serve the cranium. Although these are part of the peripheral nervous system, it's worth mentioning them here.

The cerebellum is the smaller lobe that sits at the lower back of the brain. This structure is responsible for your voluntary movements, including posture, equilibrium, and balance. It coordinates with the cerebrum to let it know if you're off balance so you can adjust accordingly.

The small brain stem, positioned at the base of the brain, is the part that connects to the spinal cord. It consists of three sections; the midbrain, the medulla oblongata, and the pons. It is responsible for many involuntary movements in your body, such as breathing, heartbeat, and digestion. It relays sensory information, controls the motion of the eyes and mouth, and directs chewing, swallowing, and vomiting. Ten more nerve pairs originate or terminate here in structures called nuclei. The brain stem has several clusters called nuclei that will be important to our understanding of the vagus nerve. In this sense, these clusters are a collection of many connecting cell bodies in the central nervous system. Remember the palm, in the hand metaphor, is the thick cell body, and a nucleus is a collection of many of those thick parts of the cells, shaking hands as if to greet each other. Those dense structures gathered together in one place cause a bulge in the nerve pathways.

Below the brain stem is the spinal cord—a multitude of nerves that travel the length of our spine within the vertebrae. Thirty-one pairs of peripheral nerves enter or exit this column. The reflex response occurs entirely within the spinal cord, rather than going to the brain.

These components of the central nervous system are all very complicated and have many more structures within them. Still, for this book, we'll leave it at this for now.

The Peripheral Nervous System

Once the nerves have traveled away from the central nervous system, they are said to be peripheral nerves. The peripheral nervous system is peripheral; in other words, it extends from the central nervous system to the outer edges of our body and everywhere in between. It consists of the 12 pairs of cranial nerves and 31 pairs of spinal nerves mentioned above. The spinal nerves leave the spinal cord via joints in the vertebrae and traverse the legs and arms, muscles and skin, bones and joints, etc. These nerves are crucial for movement, posture, muscle tone, and sensory perception.

The cranial nerves exit from the brain. Two exit from the cerebrum and the other ten exit from the brain stem. They originate or terminate in the brain stem's nuclei mentioned above. They mostly serve the brain, ears, eyes, nose, mouth, and throat, which makes them essential for seeing, hearing, tasting, smelling, chewing, swallowing, and speaking. Most of these twelve nerves emerge and remain right in the skull, which is why they are called cranial nerves. The cranial nerves all have names, but they are also numbered in descending order using Roman numerals. The first two, emerging from the cerebrum, are cranial nerves one and two (CN I and CN II). The first one arising from the brain stem is cranial nerve three (CN III), and so on. The nerves within the peripheral nervous system still may form connections in various locations. Those connections, referred to in the central nervous system as nuclei, are now called ganglions. You can identify as a bulge in the nerve.

Both the spinal nerves and the cranial nerves are all classified depending on their direction and connection. The general visceral efferent (GVE) nerves are out-going nerves that provide motor stimulation to the smooth muscles associated with visceral organs and glands. The general visceral afferent (GVA) nerves are in-coming nerves bringing sensory impulses of pain or reflex from the visceral organs, glands, and blood vessels. The special visceral afferent (SVA) nerve is a small classification of fibers that only carry smell and taste sensations to the brain. The special visceral efferent (SVE) nerve is another small classification of fibers that solely provide stimulation to the pharynx region in humans. The general somatic afferent (GSA) nerves carry sensations of pain, touch, and temperature from surface receptors throughout the body. They carry them to the central nervous system. They also carry feelings from muscles, tendons, and joints. There are a few other types of nerves, but these are the ones that are important for this book. The term, innervate, is used to describe that a nerve is serving a particular area. So, for example, the SVA fibers innervate taste buds.

Functions of the Nervous System

So, we've just taken a brief look at the relevant structures contained in the central and peripheral nervous systems. Now let's look at the functions. There are two main functions of the nervous system; the higher functions and the basic functions.

The Higher and Basic Functions

The *higher* functions separate us as humans from many of the other animals, and occur mostly in the cerebrum; things like cognition, emotions, and consciousness. Cognition is the broad term for higher thinking, including problem-solving, learning, memory storage, and retrieval, language acquisition, goal setting, self-discipline, etc. Emotions are, of course, the feelings we have. Feelings such as the joy and sorrow and amusement, love, hope, and other meaningful sentiments that make our existence worth living. Consciousness is probably the least understood function of the nervous system, but it means our understanding of who we are as individuals; our sense of self. These three functions affect and are affected by each other in a multitude of ways. They all work together to give each one of us our unique personality.

The *basic* functions of the nervous system include the somatic nervous system and the autonomic nervous system. These are the functions we share with all the other animals on our beloved little planet. The somatic nervous system, also called the voluntary nervous system because we can control many of these functions. These are motor functions that move the striated muscles that move the skeleton and sensory functions that receive information about the world within us and around us. The autonomic nervous system involves senses and actions that we can't usually control. This system senses and moves the smooth muscles of the lungs, heart, and digestive system. We'll look more at these functions next.

The Autonomic Nervous System

The autonomic nervous system involves functions that we don't have to think about, such as breathing, heartbeat, digestion, etc. These functions can be broken down even further into the sympathetic nervous system (SNS) and the parasympathetic nervous system (PNS).

The sympathetic nervous system responds to stimuli and reacts through nerves in the spinal cord. We have very little conscious control over it. It is a stress reaction that speeds up our breathing, increases our heart rate, dilates our pupils, and inhibits digestion. It also pumps noradrenaline and adrenaline into the synapses so that electrical impulses travel lightning-fast, enabling us to react quickly and survive. We call this our "fight or flight" response.

The parasympathetic nervous system has the opposite response. It slows down our heart rate and breathing while speeding up our digestive process. It also floods the synapses with the neurotransmitter acetylcholine. We call this response "rest and digest," and we also have very little conscious control over it, although it is possible to hack into it, which is the point of this whole book.

Together, the two systems are like the yin and yang of our body, each being critical under certain situations. Ideally, we should spend most of our everyday lives in the rest and digest state where we are under relatively little stress. Unfortunately, in our busy world, many of us spend more time in the fight or flight state than we should. This anxiety is what causes many of the health problems that we'll address more in Chapters 11 and 12. For now, though, let's look more closely at the structures and functions of the parasympathetic nervous system and, to be more exact, the vagus nerve in this next chapter.

CHAPTER 2

What Is the Vagus Nerve?

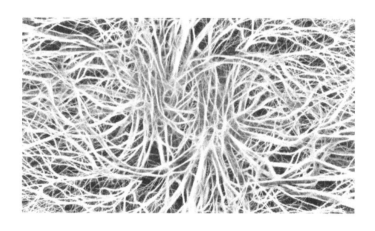

The vagus nerve is also known as cranial nerve number ten (CN X). It originates or terminates, depending on the fibers' direction, at four nuclei within the brain stem. These are the trigeminal nucleus, the nucleus tractus of solitarius, the nucleus ambiguus, and the dorsal motor nucleus of the vagus. The vagus nerve controls the body's metabolic balance, known as homeostasis. It makes sure all the internal organs are functioning correctly to keep you alive and healthy. It does this by serving as a direct line of communication between your organs and your brain, reporting problems to the brain, relaying instructions to the organs. The vagus nerve is your body's middle manager.

The vagus nerve is a bundle of five distinct types of nerve fibers. It is referred to as if it were singular though; i.e., vagus nerve instead of vagus nerves. It is aptly named "vagus" because, in Latin, "vagus" means "wandering." Think of the words vague, vagabond, or vagrant, which should give a distinct picture of how difficult it is to pin down the nerve's structure and function. Without trying to be too vague, though, as mentioned above, this nerve meanders all over the upper body and is our longest cranial nerve. It enters and exits a portion of the brain stem called the medulla oblongata on both the left and right sides through holes called the jugular foramen. So, there is a left vagus nerve and a right vagus nerve which run parallel to each other along the head and neck but go different routes once they reach the chest. At the jugular foramen, the vagus nerve traverses through two ganglia. The first ganglion is called the superior jugular ganglion, and the second one is called the inferior nodose ganglion. The vagus nerve then wanders down the neck from the brain stem, around the chest, and throughout the abdomen.

As mentioned, the vagus nerve is one of twelve pairs of cranial nerves that all work together in somatic (voluntary) and autonomic (involuntary) capacities. Most of the cranial nerves just innervate the region of the head. Yet, the vagus nerve innervates the head, the neck, the chest, and the abdomen. It is a mixed nerve because 20% of it contains afferent fibers, including the general somatic fibers, general visceral fibers, and special visceral fibers. The other 80% is efferent fibers (also remember: efferent means exiting the central nervous system), including the general visceral fibers and special visceral fibers. The vagus nerve controls 80% of our parasympathetic nervous system, so it is a significant player in our rest and digest response. There have been many exciting studies on the vagus nerve lately. These studies have led to some exciting findings on just how much it controls our lives and how much we can control it. In this chapter, we'll explore the parasympathetic pathways of the vagus nerve, where their paths originate and wander to, and what they do.

The General Visceral Efferent Pathway of the Vagus Nerve

The first type of nerve fiber in the vagus nerve that we'll explore is the general visceral efferent (GVE) fiber. It is the most complicated. It is a parasympathetic fiber that originates in the dorsal nucleus of the vagus on the left and right sides of the brain stem, coursing down both sides of the neck to the chest region. It has a minor branch along the way called the recurrent laryngeal nerve that innervates the esophagus, causing contractions that push food down toward the stomach. It also innervates the trachea causing secretion and restriction. This branch loops down on the left side around the aorta before reaching its destination at the larynx. The right recurrent vagus nerve also bends down. Yet, it slips around the right subclavian artery before returning to the larynx.

The first three major branches of the GVE pathway innervate the heart through the superior and inferior cervical cardiac nerves. The thoracic branch splits from the main nerve just above the aorta. These three branches form the cardiac plexus (a plexus is a specific area innervated by several different types of nerves). They are responsible for slowing down the rhythm of the heart, lessening the force of the beats, and lowering blood pressure. The right vagus nerve innervates the sinoatrial (SA) node, known as the heart's pacemaker. This node keeps the beat steady and reliable when functioning normally. There are so many nerves in this plexus that some people refer to it as another brain.

Next, the GVE pathway innervates the lungs with the pulmonary plexus. It is responsible for the contraction and restriction of the lungs as well as the secretion of mucus. When you're resting and relaxing, the airways don't need to be especially open since breathing tends to be shallow. A common misconception is that the vagus nerve controls the diaphragm, which controls breathing. Quite the opposite is the truth. Although the vagus nerve does go through that powerful muscle, it is the diaphragm that can control it. It is the one weapon we have to hijack the parasympathetic nervous system. With breathing techniques, we can intentionally bring calm into our being—more on this in later chapters.

The esophageal plexus is the next stop for this nerve. The esophagus continues to push food along down toward the stomach. Remember, the parasympathetic system is rest and digest. It is actively revving up the digestive organs while simultaneously slowing down the cardiac and pulmonary organs.

After the esophageal plexus, the gastric branches innervate the stomach. They cause it to mix and churn and release digestive enzymes.

The right and left vagus nerves take differing paths at this point and split off into a multitude of branches. The right GVE pathway comes from behind the esophagus to form the posterior vagal trunk. It provides most of the celiac plexus fibers, which branches off to the pancreas, the spleen, the kidneys, the adrenal gland, and the small and large intestine. There are so many nerves in this area that it is also said to be another brain. All of these organs become charged up to aid in digestion through peristalsis and enzyme secretion. The spleen and intestines are also very important in immune response and inflammation control.

The left vagus nerve swings around to the front of the esophagus and forms the anterior vagal trunk. At this point, it splits off to the hepatic plexus. This left vagus nerve provides most of the fibers to the hepatic plexus, which serves the liver by stimulating the production of glycogenesis and bile and the gallbladder by stimulating contractions to release the bile. The liver is also functional in the immune response and inflammation control.

The General Visceral Afferent Pathway of the Vagus Nerve

The general visceral afferent (GVA) fibers of the vagus nerve are sensory fibers from the same regions described above in the parasympathetic GVE pathway. They follow the same route but in the opposite direction. The GVA fibers provide sensations (usually pain, discomfort, or reflex sensations) from the internal organs, glands, and blood vessels of the abdominal, chest, and neck regions. This nerve's destination is the nucleus solutarius in the medulla oblongata. GVA fibers communicate feelings of fullness and expansion from the stomach and intestines to the brain, as well as emptiness and hunger. Recent research has suggested that the microbiome population in the gut uses the GVA pathway to cause cravings for the types of foods needed by those populations. Unhealthy cravings are why it's essential to make sure you have the healthy microbiome populations living in your intestines rather than the harmful types. If you tend always to crave sugar and highly processed foods, this might be worth a look. These fibers can also detect inflammation. The information can be used by the GVE pathway to control it. Inflammation, although good in certain situations, is very problematic when allowed to get out of control. The inflammation response will be explored further in Chapter 10.

There are three more vagal pathways, but they are part of the somatic nervous system, and we will look into them in the next chapter.

CHAPTER 3

The Role of the Vagus Nerve in the Voluntary Nervous System

The various structural systems within the peripheral nervous system make up the critical roles in sympathetic and parasympathetic nervous systems and voluntary functions. The vagus nerve is no different. Although most of the vagus nerve is involved in the involuntary portion of the autonomic nervous system, a small part functions in the somatic nervous system. The following three vagal pathways described below belong to the somatic nervous system.

The Special Visceral Efferent Pathway of the Vagus Nerve

The vagus nerve has several branches of efferent motor nerve fibers in its SVE pathway. As mentioned previously, a motor nerve serves muscles and causes them to move, sometimes voluntarily and sometimes involuntarily.

The first branch of the vagus nerve's SVE pathway is the pharyngeal nerve, which innervates most of the pharynx muscles, the soft palate, and the back of the tongue. It also causes constriction of the pharyngeal muscles to push food down towards the stomach. This nerve innervates most of the muscles in the soft palate necessary for swallowing. If something stimulates the soft palate unexpectedly or unpleasantly, the gag reflex is triggered. The gag reflex is a safety feature to prevent obstruction of the airway. The pharyngeal nerve is also the branch that innervates the Eustachian tube. When you're ascending or descending on an airplane, and you feel pressure to swallow and pop your ears, the discomfort you feel is because of uneven air pressure within those tubes. Swallowing opens them up so they can stabilize.

Just under the pharyngeal nerve is the superior laryngeal that branches again into the internal and external laryngeal branches. The internal nerve is purely sensory. We will look into it more below; however, the external nerve is exclusively motor and serves the cricothyroid muscle. This structure is responsible for pitch control of the voice by tensing and lengthening the vocal cords. Paralysis of this muscle will give you a very monotone voice.

The lowest motor branch is the recurrent laryngeal motor nerve, which innervates the larynx's remaining muscles. The recurrent laryngeal motor nerve is the primary motor supply to the muscles of the vocal cords. Vocal cords are adjusted when muscles lengthen and stretch them. As you force air through the vocal cords, different sounds are produced depending on the stretch's tension. This branch also causes the vocal folds to close when swallowing. The folding of the vocal cords is another safety feature to prevent food and liquids from entering the larynx. A third safety feature to prevent choking is the epiglottis, the flap of cartilage just above the larynx. The flap itself doesn't move, but rather, the entire larynx moves up to meet it as you swallow. When they meet, the larynx is effectively closed off.

The Special Visceral Afferent Pathway of the Vagus Nerve

The internal laryngeal nerve, branching off the superior laryngeal, as mentioned above, is purely sensory. It is the special visceral afferent (SVA) pathway of certain taste sensations from the back of the tongue and the epiglottis. This area is sensitive to the feelings of water, salt, and sour, but less likely to notice bitter and sweet. Its destination is the nucleus ambiguus, also in the medulla oblongata. Studies done on deceased animals have shown that plant-eaters have quite a few taste buds on the epiglottis.

In contrast, omnivores and carnivores have very few. People have suggested that bulky vegetation may provide more of a choking hazard, which is why herbivores need to be more sensitive in the epiglottis region, as that is the structure that covers the windpipe to prevent asphyxiation. Fewer human studies have occurred, but as expected since we are omnivores, we only have a few taste buds in the laryngeal area.

The General Somatic Afferent Pathway of the Vagus Nerve

There are two branches of the vagus nerve's GSA pathway: the auricular and the meningeal branches. The auricular branch originates in the tympanic cavity, the tympanic membrane, the external acoustic meatus, the skin in the concha of the ear, and a patch of skin behind the ear. It is also called Arnold's nerve after the German anatomist, Philipp Friedrich Arnold, discovered it in the 1800s. Another name for it is alderman's nerve because councilmen, called aldermen, would wiggle their finger in their ear when they overate. They believed stimulating the ear would help with digestion. It may, or it may not help with digestion, but it's possible since the vagus nerve connects to both the ear and the stomach. Also, when some people tickle their auricular nerve, it may cause a cough reflex.

Recent studies have shown that stimulation of this nerve can reduce some of the effects of aging, curb epileptic seizures, reduce depression, and control inflammation. A fascinating new branch of alternative medicine is opening up around this tiny section of the ear. The FDA has approved several treatments involving this auricular stimulation, and they are still discovering many other therapies. Auricular stimulation will be discussed more in later chapters.

The meningeal branch originates in the meninges, which is the tissue surrounding, cushioning, and protecting the brain. When this tissue becomes inflamed due to stress, injury, or infection, the meningeal branch will let you know with a resounding headache.

The meningeal layer is the tissue being affected when someone has meningitis.

The fibers from both of these branches have cell bodies that meet in the superior ganglion with axons that enter the skull through the jugular foramen and reach the trigeminal nucleus medulla oblongata.

CHAPTER 4

Vagus Nerve Troubles

With all these systems and organs in the body being affected by the vagus nerve, it is no wonder that the dysfunction of the nerve can lead to a plethora of problems. If you have had any chronic health problems that haven't been treatable, perhaps the vagus nerve is the source of the dysfunction and the path to healing. But how does the vagus nerve become compromised? Actually, there are several things that could damage the efficiency of the vagus nerve. Sometimes the vagus nerve is pinched between the first and second vertebrae due to injury or age. Other times the vagus nerve is severed, accidentally or intentionally, during an accident or surgery. Also, the neurotransmissions can be compromised if you are missing the necessary nutrients. Too much stress can shut it down. Chronic conditions, for example, diabetes or alcoholism, can impair the vagus nerve. The growth of a tumor can impinge on the nerve. The list goes on. It can be quite stress-ful to imagine all the ways your anti-stress system can become stressed!

As with any nerve in the body, accidents can hap-pen that will cause physical damage, deterioration, or dysfunction. The vagus nerve is no different and, being so widespread, is relatively vulnerable.

Levi* was a typical college student, playing inter-mural football, when he dove for a snag, fell, and severely broke his right scapula. Although Levi did-n't realize it at the time, the fall also impacted his first and second vertebrae causing structural insta-bility. Although this misalignment pinched his va-gus nerve, neither Levi nor his doctor realized it at the time. His doctor repaired his broken scapula, but they ignored the stiff neck he felt due to the slight cervical deviation. They assumed it was the radiating pain from the break.

Over time, Levi began experiencing other difficul-ties. First, he developed severe constipation that rendered him in constant abdominal discomfort, only being able to eliminate once every few weeks. The GI doctor gave him stool relaxers to relieve himself, but they didn't work well or consistently. He stopped eating because of his discomfort and lost a significant amount of weight. Once a six-foot-tall, 150-pound athlete, he shrunk to 104 pounds and was alarmingly thin. H barely had the energy to make it to class each day.

His grades suffered because he suddenly had a hard time thinking clearly. He had to concentrate extremely hard to comprehend the simplest of notes, read them, and re-read them into the late hours every night. Levi had always maintained an A average, but fear of a dropping grade point average caused anxiety, which didn't help his brain fog or concentration.

Levi's heart rate began to drop alarmingly low. It became normal for his resting heart rate to be in the upper 20s. He experienced dizziness and shortness of breath, which added to his lethargy and anxiety. Levi's metabolism became so sluggish that it affected even his blood cell production. He developed pancytopenia, a condition where all his blood cell types were too low.

Miraculously, Levi was able to graduate from college. Still, his poor health forced him to return home rather than embark on a career like his classmates. He spent the following two years searching for traditional medical relief from all his symptoms. He became more and more discouraged with each doctor's partial diagnosis. Not one doctor understood what was wrong with him, and each doctor treated the systems that he or she specialized in with very little success.

Eventually, Levi gave up seeing doctors and resigned himself to a life of physical suffering. He decided to concentrate on the things he could control, such as his faith, a healthy diet, steady exercise, and calming techniques. With youth and time on his side, Levi began to improve very slowly. He became less anxious about his symptoms and started getting on with his life, eventually going back to school for his master's degree.

The body is a fantastic machine that will heal itself, given half a chance. Levi's symptoms, in hindsight, were clearly all related to pressure on the vagus nerve. Once the pressure from the initial injury eventually subsided, all the symptoms went gradually away as well. Had the root cause of the problems been discovered right away, years of suffering could have been alleviated.

As with Levi, sometimes, the vagus nerve can become pinched between the vertebrae. A branch of holistic medicine has revolved around healing the vagus nerve at its source. This remedy involves straightening out the cervical spine after an accident or normal wear and tear with age, so that the vagus nerve is no longer under pressure. The exact location of the stress and its severity can lead to many problems that range from gastrointestinal distress to dizziness to an irregular heartbeat, speech problems, and even depression. These symptoms could all occur at once and seem utterly unrelated if no one could find the cause. A person who is suffering from this might have five different doctors, treating each symptom with different medications, and not communicating at all.

Another malady caused possibly by pressure from the vertebrae is Meniere's disease (MD). This disease was first identified in the early 1800s by Prosper Ménière, a French doctor who first identified a combination of symptoms in the inner ear. Episodes of vertigo, tinnitus (ringing in the ear), progressive hearing loss, and feelings of fullness in the ear can occur in spells, leaving the person feeling as if the world is spinning. If left unchecked, Meniere's disease can lead to permanent loss of hearing. Many doctors don't agree on the cause of this disease, however recent studies have shown a link between it and cervical instability because of whiplash. If the brain stem and associated nerves, including the vagus nerve, are impinged or crushed because of pressure from the cervical vertebrae, symptoms can appear gradually within a month of the accident. A 2017 study, "Vagus Nerve Stimulation Paired with Tones for the Treatment of Tinnitus: A Prospective Randomized Double-blind Controlled Pilot Study in Humans" by Richard Tyler, Anthony Cacace, Christina Stocking, et al., showed treatments involving the vagal nerve had had a positive effect on participants in the study in the relief of tinnitus symptoms.

Another possible way for the vagus nerve to become damaged is during surgery. When a patient has cysts, a goiter, Grave's disease, or cancer, they may need to have surgery to remove some or even all of their thyroid. Due to individual anatomical differences, though, the external arm of the superior laryngeal branch of the vagus nerve is sometimes accidentally severed. Severing this nerve will permanently disable the cricothyroid muscle, the muscle responsible for pitch and voice projection. Even more problematic, the inferior laryngeal branch of the vagus nerve, responsible for most of the larynx muscles, can sometimes be accidentally severed. If the inferior laryngeal branch is severed, it can cause chronic hoarseness, difficulty swallowing, and acute airway obstruction. Finally, your doctor could also accidentally cut your recurrent laryngeal branch of the vagus nerve during thyroid surgery. Consequent symptoms from this can include hoarseness, acute airway obstruction, and changes to the patient's voice. Differences in sound production is an especially unfortunate situation for individuals who use their voices professionally.

Cindy* was a talented singer who aspired to sing professionally in the opera. She majored in voice in college and had taken years of voice lessons. She was plagued though by cysts on her thyroid and decided that the best course of action was to remove the problematic portion. Tragically, during the operation, the recurrent laryngeal branch of her vagus nerve was nicked. This accident caused just enough damage to end her singing career before it ever had a chance to launch.

Sometimes, people with extreme obesity or severe peptic stomach ulcers elect to have their vagus nerve cut intentionally. This procedure, called a vagotomy, was once a fairly standard procedure for these maladies. It required a week's stay in the hospital. The nerve was cut entirely above the stomach, and once cut, there was no possibility of repair. This maneuver reduced the amount of stomach acid that the patient could secrete into the stomach. It also eliminated hunger sensations. It did have some unpleasant side effects, though, such as diarrhea, vomiting, cramping, bloating, flushing, dizziness, and compromised immunity.

Now, although less used, the procedure is much more refined. Doctors will now only cut branches of the nerve that lead to the stomach so that the vagus nerve can innervate the other abdominal organs. Researchers are exploring different, even less drastic procedures are that simply block the signals using electrical impulses. Many people have reported significant weight loss using these techniques.

Doug* was over three hundred pounds when he heard about the procedure. He had tried everything to lose weight but just couldn't keep the pounds off. Staples and stomach reduction surgery had too many complications, and Doug simply didn't want to take those risks. The partial vagotomy appealed to him, so he decided to give it a try. Within months of the procedure, Doug lost upwards of 60 pounds. A year later, with exercise and a sensible diet, he lost 40 more pounds. Chewing slowly and savoring each bite, Doug says that he enjoys food more now. Doug is never starving, so he can afford to take his time rather than gobbling his dinner as he did before.

Another issue for the vagus nerve is when it becomes irritated. So, what causes the vagus nerve to get irritated? Gastrointestinal distress can put pressure on the nerve and hurt it, with a hiatal hernia being one of the most likely culprits. A hiatal hernia occurs because of injury or heavy lifting. It causes the upper portion of the stomach to slip up through the diaphragm and into the chest region. The stomach's pressure squeezing through the opening in the diaphragm that the vagus nerve also goes through, puts undue constriction on the nerve. Poor posture, spicy foods, and even stress can also inflame the nerve, along with anxiousness and exhaustion. Tumors can grow almost anywhere. If one happens to grow near the vagus nerve, crowding it and impeding its path like the hernia, symptoms similar to many of the ones described above may arise.

Jenny* was suffering from a variety of conditions that seemed to engulf her all at once. She experienced abdominal bloating, burping, heartburn, diarrhea, irregular heartbeat, and shortness of breath. Her heart doctor had ruled out heart disease, and her gut doctor had found nothing remarkable on her endoscopy. She was seeing a dietitian and was taking antacids for her gas and reflux. She couldn't help thinking that it was too coincidental to have gone from having no symptoms to having all of these symptoms. She believed there had to be a connection. She decided, with the help of her dietitian, to switch to a strict anti-inflammatory diet. She cut out all sugar, processed grains, unhealthy fats, dairy, and processed meats. She also began to seek acupuncture to relieve the inflammation and yoga to calm her vagus nerve. After just a few weeks, Jenny began to feel significantly better. She continues to choose her food wisely, maintains a regular yoga practice, and receives acupuncture as needed.

Mast cell activation syndrome is one chronic condition caused by an overactive vagus nerve. White blood cells are active members of the body's protection from external invasives. While most white blood cells are suspended in the blood, mast cells are white blood cells that are fixed to certain types of tissue. Mast cell activation syndrome (MCAS) is a condition where the mast cells release too much of a chemical that causes anaphylaxis, or near-anaphylaxis, type symptoms. These symptoms include rash, itchiness, lightheadedness, diarrhea, nausea, vomiting, shortness of breath, difficulty breathing, difficulty swallowing, and congestion. A 2006 study, Stead RH, Colley EC, Wang B, et al. Vagal influences over mast cells, links this syndrome with vagus dysfunction.

Yet another vagus nerve malady is neuropathy. People with insulin-dependent diabetes or alcoholism can develop neuropathy in many nerves, and the vagus nerve is no exception. The long-term exposure to toxic chemicals in the blood eventually wear away at the myelin sheath, the protective coating surrounding the cell's axons. Neuropathy causes unexplainable pain and sensitivity, as well as a loss of muscle control. The most common symptom of vagal neuropathy is gastroparesis. Gastroparesis is a condition where the stomach's food remains there too long because it isn't adequately churned and digested. Gastroparesis is a painful condition with no cure, and can you only treat it with lifestyle changes? Its symptoms include acid reflux, vomiting, bloating, cramping, and diarrhea.

One more example of a condition resulting from a compromised vagus nerve is postural orthostatic tachycardia syndrome (POTS). POTS is an out of control heart rate increase of 30 beats per minute or more, or above 120 beats per minute, within the first 10 minutes of standing, without a drop in blood pressure. Symptoms associated with POTS include heart irregularity, exercise intolerance, lightheadedness, tremor, nausea, fainting, headache, and fatigue. Chronic fatigue syndrome (CFS) is often a comorbidity of POTS. A 2019 study, Jacob G, Diedrich L, Sato K, et al. Vagal and Sympathetic Function in Neuropathic Postural Tachycardia Syndrome, linked this syndrome to poor vagus functioning.

For the vagus nerve to function correctly and efficiently, acetylcholine must be present in the synapses between the nerves and their targets. Acetylcholine is the isotope that carries the electrical impulse across the synaptic space. Without enough of it in your system, the neurons will be transferring information slower than they should. Unfortunately, you can't just go out and eat the stuff. Your body must make it. The B complex vitamins are necessary for making the acetyl group. B complex vitamins can be taken in the form of supplements or eating grass-fed meats, dairy, eggs, whole grains, legumes, and green leafy vegetables. You can find choline in grass-fed meats and eggs. Maintaining a diet rich in these foods will help maintain vitality so your vagus nerve can perform optimally.

The most widespread disorder associated with the vagus nerve is inflammation. The vagus nerve communicates closely with the liver, the spleen, and the intestines, all active in the immune response when signal proteins are detected anywhere in the body. Unfortunately, the response gets confused between invading cells and the body's cells. This confusion leads to chronic inflammation, which opens the Pandora's Box of maladies. Chronic inflammation is responsible for heart disease, diabetes, Alzheimer's, Crohn's disease, cancer, rheumatoid arthritis, just to name a few. We will address much more on these conditions in later chapters.

When a person's vagus nerve is structurally sound and functioning well, they are said to have a healthy vagal tone. A healthy vagal tone is associated with an optimistic outlook, secure social networking, and good health. One of the best ways to measure vagal tone is heart rate variation (HRV). A person with a high HRV has a healthy vagal tone. Someone with a low HRV has a poor vagal tone.

Although a healthy vagal tone is undoubtedly desirable, it is possible to have an overactive vagus nerve. The overactive vagus nerve will show symptoms of bradycardia (a slow heart rate), shortness of breathing, obesity, diabetes, diarrhea, congestion, and fainting. When the vagus nerve is overactive, normal daily functions such as laughter, urination, swallowing, coughing, or even pooping can cause fainting.

The vegas nerve is supposed to reduce stress; too much stress, however, overloads the system. If left too long in the fight or flight state, the vagus nerve will stop trying to override it and just accept those adrenaline levels as standard. This situation causes the vagus nerve to become underactive. An underactive vagus nerve has symptoms of heartburn, constipation or diarrhea, gas and bloating, inflammation, infections, stress, accelerated or irregular heart rate, high blood pressure, dizziness, brain fog, problems swallowing, and an unsteady voice. When the vagus nerve is underactive, it is called a poor vagal tone. Strokes, heart attacks, loneliness, depression, and negativity are conditions that are also associated with a poor vagal tone. What causes a poor vagal tone? Any of the above physical problems can create a poor vagal tone. Still, there are chemical and physiological reasons as well. Avoiding stressful situations, eating a healthy diet, and resetting your vagal tone will help you return to a healthy functioning level.

*Names have been changed to protect the identities of individuals. In some cases, the stories of a few individuals with similar details have been merged into one account.

CHAPTER 5

How the Vagus Nerve Controls Breathing and How the Vagus Nerve System Helps Make Memories

Cases of Alzheimer's and dementia are on the rise, and frankly, it's disturbing. If you've ever spent time with a loved one who has forgotten who you are, you know how painful it is. Conversely, maybe you worry about forgetting the names of your loved ones. Imagine how terrifying it might be to wake up every morning in an unfamiliar place, with strange people who seem to expect something from you. It's hard even to imagine how frustrating and even frightening that would be. Because of this rise in memory loss, there has been substantial research done in recent years, and there have been some surprising findings.

Not that long ago, people assumed that dementia was a natural part of growing older. People thought

Alzheimer's was strictly hereditary, and you either got it or you didn't. Either way, they were considered to be unavoidable. However, it is becoming more apparent that individual lifestyle choices can postpone, or even avoid, the devastating effects of memory loss. Some of those lifestyle choices include eating right and exercising, getting plenty of sleep, avoiding toxins like cigarette smoke and alcohol, and maintaining healthy relationships.

But here's a surprise; you need to make memories before you even need to worry about losing them. Sure, that doesn't sound so profound, but people often leave it out of the equation. Perhaps this is why mindfulness has suddenly become so popular. If you are always in a constant state of distraction, you may not be aware of the things you'll wish you remembered. If you are mindful, though, you'll make memories worth keeping.

Being mindful involves being aware of the present moment by using all your senses. Wherever you are, whatever you're doing, what do you see? What colors are surrounding you? How many shades of brown can you count? What's the most predominant color? I've never noticed this before, but looking up from my computer right now, I'm suddenly aware of all the yellow in my workspace. My wall is a lion yellow, my post-it notes and notepad are a pale yellow, the light from my lamp is a warm yellow, there's a bowl of lemons that are a lemon yellow. Furthermore, my lava lamp is a greenish-yellow, and some packages are a brownish-orangey yellow. I have never noticed that there were so many yellows at my workspace.

Next, what do you hear? I just heard thunder; my dog is snoring, my computer is making tiny clicking noises, some Sandhill cranes are calling. Wait, my dog just walked by. That must have been my cat snoring.

Touch? What do you feel? I feel the warmth of my computer keys, the ache in my neck from looking down at my computer, and the firm chair on which I'm sitting. The room is a little chilly, so my arms feel a slight chill.

Taste? Are you eating or drinking anything? Is it salty or sweet? Can you identify more than one flavor in your mouth at once? Is it exciting or comforting? Or do you like it at all?

How about the smells? On what fragrances are you able to focus? Take a deep breath through your nose and pay attention to any scents you have been ignoring until now. You may not even be conscious of smelling anything, but breathing through your nose, has helped you form memories. Yep, it's true. Recent studies are finding that breathing through your nose is beneficial to making memories. Wait; what? That's right. Current studies are finding that breathing through your nose is useful for making memories regardless of any scents being present.

According to a Journal of Neuroscience 2016 study by Zelano et al., breathing through the nose coordinates with the electrical activity in the brain. Their findings showed that brain waves peaked while subjects were breathing through their nose, and the brain waves reduced while the participants breathed through their mouths. More specifically, the experiments identified the brain activity to be fear discrimination and memory retrieval. Maybe you've noticed that smells have a unique way of bringing back profoundly poignant memories. There is something to that, but this study found that nose breathing, even without the stimulation of scent, is a significantly more reliable way to make and retrieve memories. Zelano's research found that test subjects could recognize facial expressions faster, especially fearful expressions if the participants were inhaling through their nose. Test subjects in another study were able to remember random objects better while inhaling. In both tests, the results were negative when the participants were breathing through their mouths.

In another study in The Journal of Neuroscience, by Karolinska Institute in Sweden, similar findings were reported. This time, researchers had the test subjects breathe through their nose for one hour after learning twelve different smells. They repeated the test with twelve more scents after breathing through their mouth for one hour. Then they were presented with aromas that were from either group or even new smells. The participants were able to identify the odors that they learned before nose breathing the most successfully.

Breathing Problems During Sleep Linked to Memory Problems, a study reported in WebMD 2011, showed just what the title suggests. They compared 298 women with sleep-disordered breathing problems who had an average age of 82. After five years, they examined the participants again. The results showed that 45% of the women with sleep-disordered breathing had developed memory problems compared with 31% of women without the disorder. Interestingly, contrary to typical advice, neither the number of times their sleep was disrupted, nor the number of hours they slept were associated with the risk. Breathing through the nose, and therefore oxygen levels during sleep, were deemed the primary culprit for whether memory problems would become an issue. There are effective treatments for sleep-disordered breathing, so take heart if this describes you, and seek help.

So how do these discoveries relate to the vagus nerve? The vagus nerve is the coordinator for calming you down, slowing your breathing, and lowering your heart rate, among other things. The response will naturally happen as you relax, but you can also flip it yourself by controlling your breathing. To control your breathing, you need to engage your diaphragm and take in a deep, slow breath through your nose, hold it briefly, and then release your breath for a slightly longer duration than you drew it in. This practice will bring about an almost immediate sense of calm. Why is calm important to memory? Education knows.

The field of education has had an about-face in the past 30 years. While once educators were encouraged to keep the students quiet, in line, and afraid to interrupt, now they are taught to make the classroom friendly, involved, and even playful. Why? So, students will feel calm and happy and safe. Research now shows that students learn and also retain information better when they are comfortable and not worried about physical and emotional needs. If students qualify financially, food is given to them, if they don't qualify financially, food is available to them. Counselors are accessible to students so they can talk through problems. Social workers help students with family problems. Teachers are on the front line to get to know each student and make them feel welcome. Schools do not tolerate bullying, and they teach students how to resolve conflicts in a non-violent way. All this is so that the school environment will be a happy place and conducive to learning. Safety equals calm; calm equals open; open equals learning; and learning equals memory formation. Now we're back to the vagus nerve.

We can't always control our environment. We try to control it for our children at home and in school, but we aren't necessarily able to do the same for ourselves. We often can't help the situations in which we find ourselves. Our only alternative is to choose calm despite the chaos, especially in a dangerous circumstance.

Juanita* was a faithful practitioner of yoga. She'd injured her neck years ago in a diving accident. She had no alternative but to do yoga daily to relieve the pain and maintain her range of motion. She knew there were other benefits to yoga, but those weren't why she was faithful to the art. Still, she forced herself to diligently practice all aspects of yoga, including breath body links, meditative postures, and peaceful patience with herself in each new pose.

One evening, Juanita was picking up a few groceries after her shift at the seafood restaurant, where she worked as a server. There were a few other people in the store, and she was behind most of them in line. The self-absorbed woman at the front of the line had at least a dozen coupons, and there were no other open registers. With aching feet and a sour attitude, Juanita began activating her breathing techniques from yoga to remain calm. Using her diaphragm, she discreetly but deeply inhaled through her nose: 1, 2, 3, 4. Juanita held it: 1, 2, 3, 4. Then she gently released it: 1, 2, 3, 4, 5, 6. Rather than thinking about the annoyance she felt, Juanita concentrated on being mindful as she continued her breathing.

Suddenly and very quietly, when the cashier finally opened the drawer to cash out the coupon lady, the man who was second in line calmly pulled out a gun. He told the cashier to hand over all the money in the register so that no one would get hurt. Before Juanita even realized what was happening, she was in the midst of a robbery. As panic was threatening to take over, Juanita's years of yoga stood in the way. She continued breathing in through her nose, holding briefly, letting out a bit slower. As the gunman fled with his wad of cash, the situation was over so quickly that the stunned customers and shaken cashier just looked at each other in disbelief. Seconds that felt like minutes later, a few of them had the presence of mind to call 911.

Everyone had to remain at the store, of course, for the police report, and each person gave their version of what happened. Juanita, who had been practicing her calm breathing at the time of the robbery, gave the most detailed account. Much to her tired feet's displeasure, Juanita had to stay the longest for the police's report. Her accurate recollection led to the identification of the armed robber.

Juanita's story is a prime example of how you can manipulate the vagus nerve to work for you if you have the mind to remember to use it. There are many other situations when you can enhance your memory by breathing. These situations include times such as when you are studying for a test, preparing to give a speech, showing off a magic trick, or telling a good story. Try to remain calm, breathe deeply through your nose, and stay mindful.

*Names have been changed to protect the identities of individuals. In some cases, the stories of a few individuals with similar details have been merged into one account.

CHAPTER 6

Vagal Nerve Stimulation Surgery and the Implantation of the Device

The vagus nerve, as we've seen, has pathways throughout the body that control many processes. And we've looked at many of the things that can go wrong with it. But new technology is gaining significance in using the vagus nerve and all its branches to affect many of those different systems. The FDA first approved epilepsy for this type of therapy.

Seizures can vary between bouts of violent, uncontrolled shaking and loss of consciousness to a mere loss of awareness that can last a few seconds up to a few minutes. People can have seizures because of low blood sugar, low sodium levels, withdrawal from drugs or alcohol, fever, concussion, or brain infection. Sometimes, however, seizures can be caused by an unexplained brain disorder, often resulting from injury or stroke, that causes neurons to be over-stimulated. When this becomes a recurring problem, it is known as epilepsy. Most of the time, epilepsy, which affects approximately 68 million people worldwide, is controlled by medications. People who suffer from it can lead normal lives if they remain on their medication. Medicine doesn't always work, though, on approximately 30% of the patients. Then, epilepsy can be debilitating, and patients cannot experience a healthy, satisfying life. Individuals who don't respond to medication must remain on constant alert, waiting for their next seizure. Activities such as work, school, or social outings are not possible, and driving is out of the question. Many places do not permit driving until a year has passed since the last seizure. Up until a few years ago, these people felt hopeless. In 1997, a new therapy was approved by the FDA that helped curb or even stop their seizures, allowing them to get back to the business of living.

As far back as the 1880s, researchers designed instruments used to decrease cerebral blood flow and electronically stimulate the human vagus nerve to stop seizures. The invention, by New York neurologist James Leonard Corning, was not widely accepted, however. Due to side effects such as dizziness, fainting, and an unusually slow heart rate, it wasn't well-received. In 1938 Bailey P, Bremer FA published the paper *Sensory Cortical Representation of the Vagus Nerve*. It documented that vagal stimulation caused electro-encephalogram changes. In 1951, Olson Dell showed that stimulation of the vagus nerve caused responses in regions of the thalamus. Another study done in 1985 by Zabara et al. linked vagus nerve stimulation to seizure termination in dogs. In 1988, four patients volunteered to participate in the first pilot study on a vagus nerve stimulator (VNS) implantation in humans for epilepsy. Two of the patients reported complete seizure control. One reported a 40% seizure reduction in the number of seizures, and one said there was no effect at all. Finally, in 1997, the VNS device was approved by the US Food and Drug Administration. Cyberonics, a Houston, TX-based medical supply company that has since merged to form LivaNova, created it.

The VNS device is a small coiled structure wrapped around the left vagus nerve at the throat level. The right vagus nerve innervates the heart, and stimulation could cause heart complications; therefore, doctors usually implant the device on the left side. A wire attached to the coil runs under the skin to a small, watch-sized, battery-operated pulse generator placed under the skin on the chest. Its size and concept is much like a pacemaker. Patients have the device surgically implanted on an outpatient basis. The most significant risk is an infection at the site of the incision. If for any reason, the patient would like to have the device removed, that is also a simple procedure.

Because of VNS therapy, individuals with epilepsy reported a reduction in seizures in approximately 80% of the recipients. These statistics improve the more prolonged the VNS device is in place and operating. People who have benefitted from this therapy have been able to get their lives back.

Ten years ago, Jessie* was an active teenager. Jessie enjoyed sports, hanging out with his friends, and had a part-time job. His grades in school were excellent, and Jessie was hoping for athletic and academic scholarships to college. He wanted to get a degree in computer programming and was excited about his future. Jessie was involved in church and went on mission trips every summer. He was the life of every social gathering because his energy and joy were contagious. Nothing embarrassed him because Jessie was so comfortable with himself; he was open and honest and real. He loved karaoke even though he couldn't sing very well at all. It didn't matter, though. He seized every day as if it were his last and looked at every challenge as if it were an adventure.

Then, tragically, Jessie was involved in a head-on automobile collision on his way home from work one Saturday night. In an instant, Jessie's life changed forever. He had a head injury and was in a coma for a few days. When he woke up, he began having seizures. Suddenly, instead of him seizing every day, each day seized him. He had ten to twelve seizures every day, each lasting for up to an hour, including recovery time. He took a dozen different medications that were supposed to control the seizures but had minimal effect. Once so optimistic about their son's future, his parents lives now revolved around his health care, and they became his only companions. His mom had to quit her job just to stay home and care for him. Jessie could no longer attend school because his seizures were so disruptive and even potentially dangerous. He was confined to his home, no longer able to enjoy the freedom of driving, the satisfaction of earning his paycheck, the hope of going on to college. His friends came to visit him regularly at first. Eventually, though, they moved on with their own lives, going off to college, getting married, joining the military.

Jessie sank into depression. The daily drudgery of taking all those medications to no avail wore on his, once indefatigably, bright outlook. The side effects were almost as adverse as the seizures themselves. He gained weight, felt dizzy, lost hope. His parents' lives centered on taking turns caring for him, and in a very real way, they lost their lives as well.

Then, after a particularly severe seizure that led them to the emergency room for stitches, the young

ER doctor asked them if they had ever heard of VNS therapy. It was a relatively new treatment at the time, and they had not heard of it. Desperate for help, though, they were willing to try anything. With the advice of that young doctor, they found a clinic specializing in VNS therapy and made an appointment for a consultation. Within a week, they sat in an examining room, learning of a procedure that had the potential to change their lives entirely again. They decided to go for it.

A spark that hadn't been apparent in years began to glow in Jessie's eyes. He believed that this was the answer for which he had been waiting. His parents, however, were afraid to hope. They couldn't bear it if they had to watch their once vibrant son sink into even more profound discouragement. They tried to temper Jessie's enthusiasm with caution, reminding him that it didn't work in every case. And also, if it did help, he probably wouldn't be seizure-free. Jessie remained optimistic, though.

Three weeks after that fateful trip to the emergency room, Jessie and his parents were sitting in a waiting room, waiting for a miracle. He anxiously waited to be taken back to begin the surgical VNS procedure. Jessie's foot tapped nervously as his parents, holding hands, prayed silently for relief for their son. Finally, a nurse came for him, and he began the short one-hour procedure that would prove to be, in his case, the best decision he ever made. They gave Jessie a light anesthesia, and they slit a small incision on the left side of his neck. They wrapped a tiny coil was around his vagus nerve. Then they put another incision in his chest where they implanted a small battery-operated charging device under the tissue. They connected the two apparatuses with an imperceptible subdermal wire. Another hour of recovery time in the office and Jessie was ready to return home to begin the process of recovery.

Two weeks later, Jessie and his parents returned to the clinic, where they received operating instructions for the VNS device. The doctor set the charge generator to send small electrical surges through his vagus nerve and into his brain at regular intervals. The doctor taught Jessie and his parents how to manually release the charge if he felt a seizure coming on. In the days and weeks to come, Jessie had to return to the clinic a few times to adjust the frequency and strength of the electrical charge to meet Jessie's personal needs, but there were signs of hope. The severity of his seizures began to diminish, and eventually, the frequency did as well. A few months ago, he had multiple, crippling seizures every day that drained him of energy and strength. Now he was having just one or two seizures each day that were barely mild enough to interrupt his activity.

Gradually, Jessie's confidence grew as he learned how to manage his VNS therapy. He began getting involved again in church activities. With his doctor's approval, he lessened the number of medications he was on, which, in turn, eased him of the unpleasant side effects. He signed up to take classes online, finally having the ability to concentrate long enough to get his GED. And his family began going out to eat together, hiking in the park, and enjoying a movie again. His parents even returned to their weekly date nights. They remembered why they fell in love so many years ago, confident that they could leave Jessie alone or with friends.

That was ten years ago, and Jessie now lives a mostly healthy life. He still uses his VNS therapy device, but he barely even notices the mild, regular vibrations. When Jessie does sense it, Jessie feels comforted and grateful. He eventually got his degree in computer programming, and he now has a successful and satisfying career. Jessie can leave home without the fear of not knowing what will happen to him each day. He seizes the day again without letting it seize him. And his parents thank God every day to have their son back, to see his smile.

VNS therapy isn't right for everyone, but 80% of the patients who have tried it are experiencing benefits from it, and 73% have chosen to remain on the therapy long-term. The FDA has approved the use of VNS therapy in children as young as four years of age. Because childhood is such a critical time of growth and development, uncontrolled seizures can be permanently debilitating. With the VNS device, though, 63% of the children using it have fewer seizures, with 48% having shorter seizures.

Recently, researchers have developed and are studying a new noninvasive (nVNS) procedure. They designed it to have electrical stimulation applied across the skin just over the auricular branch of the vagus nerve. This nerve innervates the middle part of the ear and gives similar results as the invasive VNS. The electrical impulse is carried by the vagus afferent pathway back to the nucleus of the solitary tract in the brainstem. There it goes on to activate portions of the brain that control seizures. The nVNS has the advantage of not requiring surgery to implant, so there's no risk of infection. There is a portable stimulator with a digital interface that allows the user to monitor signal amplitude. Seizure frequency is reduced in 45% of the patients using it, going up to 54% after six months. Researchers need to do long-term studies to determine whether patients are dependable enough to handle the removable device consistently. If not, they may be better off having it implanted in the more permanent procedure, ensuring consistency and efficacy.

Dr. Matthew Leonard is the Assistant Professor of Neurological Surgery in the Weill Institute for Neurosciences at the University of California, San Francisco. He has been investigating nVNS' effectiveness because it's still unclear how similar nVNS is to an implanted VNS device. Leonard's team records neural activity directly from the human brain in patients with epilepsy. Some of the participants have the surgically inserted cervical VNS device. They also volunteer to wear the ear device for a few minutes. This way, researchers can see if the stimulation in the brain is similar between the two devices.

Whether it is implanted in the neck or inserted in the ear, this therapy can give profound relief to many maladies besides epilepsy. The FDA has approved it to treat depression, inflammation, and migraines. Researchers are even studying the use of nVNS to assist in language acquisition. With minimal side effects and maximum potential, nVNS therapy is on the cutting edge of a medical revolution. Researchers need to have it thoroughly explored.

*Names have been changed to protect the identities of individuals. In some cases, the stories of a few individuals with similar details have been merged into one account.

CHAPTER 7

Risks, Treatment, and the Side Effects of Vagal Nerve Stimulation

The VNS surgery itself is a one hour, outpatient, minimally invasive procedure. Risks associated with VNS are minimal. A few rare occurrences of difficulty swallowing and vocal cord paralysis are possible if there is a mishap during surgery. Coughing, pain, and labored breathing are also frequently reported. In a study on epileptic children by Zaaimi et al. in 2005 and another by Nagarajan et al. in 2003, a reduction in oxygen saturation during sleep was observed in most patients. Another study by Khurana et al. in 2007 reports stimulus-induced sleep apnea.

Other risks include injury during surgery to the vagus nerve, the vocal cords, or blood vessels nearby. The closest blood vessels are the carotid artery and the jugular vein. As with any surgery, there are bleeding, pain, and infection risks at the incision site, and possible anesthesia reactions.

A few weeks after the surgery, when the incisions have begun to heal, the patient returns to have the electrical pulse generator activated and programmed according to the patient's needs. The duration, frequency, and current can all be adjusted. Typically, the patient's stimulation begins at a low level. Gradually, the doctor will increase the electrical stimulation according to the severity of the symptoms. He will also set the stimulus to turn on and off in cyclic intervals. A thirty second on and five minutes off range is a typical setting. When the stimulation occurs, there may be a slight tingling or pain in the neck area with hoarseness until the stimulus is over.

Some newer models of VNS can detect seizure activity and activate the stimulations to prevent the seizure from worsening. A hand-held magnet also comes with the device and can be used to initiate stimulation if needed manually. It can also turn off the machine for activities such as singing or public speaking when the user doesn't want to be interrupted by hoarseness.

Newer still is a wireless VNS model. This more modern device eliminates the need for a chest incision or connecting wire. Instead, the doctor implants the much smaller charge generator in the same location as the coils around the vagus nerve. The patient must plug in the wireless charging apparatus once a week. The doctor can control the device settings via a smartphone app.

No matter what the model of VNS used, periodic visits will need to be made to the doctor to make sure the device is functioning correctly, the settings are appropriate for the symptoms, and no infection has erupted in the incision sites.

Several side effects can occur with VNS. These include voice changes, hoarseness, throat pain, cough, headaches, shortness of breath, difficulty swallowing, skin tingles, sleep apnea, and insomnia. Most patients found these side effects to be tolerable and even lessened with time.

CHAPTER 8

The Advantages of Vagal
Nerve Activation

The most significant advantage of vagal nerve activation is a higher heart rate variability (HRV).

Likewise, probably the most reliable way to determine the health of your vagal tone is to monitor your HRV. The HRV is a measure of how well your sympathetic and parasympathetic nervous systems balance each other out. The higher your HRV, the better they are balanced. If you have a poor vagal tone, the HRV will be low, meaning the sympathetic branch of your nervous system makes you work harder than you need to. This sympathetic over-activity leaves your body in a stress state with less energy to do the things you'd rather be doing. It also makes you much more susceptible to disease.

Ideally, the sympathetic nervous system and the parasympathetic nervous system work closely together to maintain health. When the body is in the fight or flight mode, the rest and digest mode is waiting in the wings to bring everything back to normal. When the body is resting and digesting, the fight or flight response is on call if an emergency occurs. As we age, we find ourselves more and more in the fight or flight response, even when there is no emergency to surmount.

Many factors determine how healthy your HRV is, such as age, activity level, nutrition, and gender. It isn't useful to compare your HRV to other people because there are so many variables. The more meaningful comparison would be to monitor your trends over time. If you are making valiant efforts to improve your vagal tone's health, you should see your HRV go up. HRV monitors are devices you can purchase to keep track of your progress. HRV will be explained more in subsequent chapters.

So how do you activate your vagus nerve to drive up your HRV? There are many ways:

✓ **Drink plenty of water.** Staying hydrated is the easiest way to have the most significant impact on your vagal tone. Being dehydrated by just 2% can affect your tone negatively.

✓ **Get quality sleep.** If you have sleep apnea or other breathing problems, seek help. There are cures for poor sleep issues. Also, if possible, sleep on your right side to stimulate your vagus nerve.

✓ **Eat whole, natural foods.** Highly processed foods are like sludge in your system. Sugar, white flour, white rice, unhealthy fats, dyes, and preservatives clean them all out and then keep them out. Don't even bring them into your house.

✓ **Know your alcohol limits and be mindful of them.** Everyone's ability to metabolize alcohol is different. And people metabolize various types of liquor differently under different circumstances. One night of irresponsible drinking can lower your vagal tone for up to 5 days. Just watch it. Better yet, don't drink alcohol at all.

✓ **Be gentle with yourself.** Get a massage, try an Epsom salt bath, take naps, meditate.

✓ **Be consistent.** Just like pets and children, your body performs better when it knows what to expect. Stick to a regular bedtime, be devoted to your workout schedule, eat meals within a daily window.

✓ **Try intermittent fasting.** The sage advice of three square meals per day is old news. The smaller your window of eating is, the more your vagus nerve will be activated. You should have a maximum eating window of twelve hours. Anything less than that is even better. Make sure you're drinking that water, though.

✓ **Build positive social networks.** Blue Zones by Dan Buettner compares areas where people live the longest. The biggest common denominator between them is strong social interaction. Making eye contact with people you like gives your parasympathetic nervous system a jolt! You can't get that from social media.

✓ **Get outside**. Connect with nature, breathing in the fresh air, soaking up some vitamin D from the sun. Do this every day, and your vagus nerve will thank you. While you're outside, take your shoes off and let the electrons from the earth flow up through your feet and into your body.

✓ **Laugh, hum, sing, dance, and play**. Joan Erikson once said, "We don't stop playing because we get old. We get old because we stop playing." Quit being so serious, lighten up, chill out, sing and hum and laugh. These activities cause a vibration that activates your vagus nerve.

✓ **Be cold**. We tend to reach for a sweater whenever we feel a slight chill. Instead, we should embrace the cooler temperatures because it wakes up the vagus nerve. Slap your face with cold water, take a cold shower, drink ice-cold water, jump in that cold stream, and keep the heater low or off. If you have a heart condition, you should be sure to consult your doctor, though, before jumping into a cold shower or stream. These activities can cause an increase in heart rate and blood pressure.

✓ **Eat seafood or take fish oil supplements.** Researchers have found that nutrients in seafood will activate the vagus nerve.

✓ **Engage your abdominal muscles.** The sensations felt while coughing or pooping are carried by the vagus nerve. Doing sit-ups or other abdominal workouts may help to activate it.

✓ **Feed and grow your micro friends.** Prebiotics, probiotics, fiber, green leafy vegetables; these will all improve your gut health, which will enhance the communications between your intestine and your brain via the vagus.

✓ **Poop daily.** Getting rid of those toxins and allowing the digestive system to move is one of the best ways to maintain your vagal tone.

✓ **Consider VNS therapy.** You may have one of the growing number of conditions that will benefit from the stimulation. If you've been suffering from epilepsy, depression, or

Crohn's disease and medication hasn't helped, see your doctor about VNS therapy. You can even purchase new nVNS devices over the internet without a prescription.

✓ **Practice yoga**. I can't say it enough, but I'll try in Chapter 16. Yoga is your vagus nerve's best friend.

✓ **Exercise**. Move. Get your circulation flowing. Sweat. Breathe. Set physical goals. Reach those goals. Set more goals. Find a workout buddy. Join a gym. Document your progress. Enter races. Take exercise classes. Whether you believe it or even if you don't, the more you exercise, the more you'll want to move. The more you are sedentary, the more you'll remain sedentary. Your body was designed for motion.

That was a pretty exhaustive list. Notice those bullets are check marks? With your doctor's approval, try to check them all off. As you incorporate more and more vagus activating habits into your lifestyle, your overall health will improve. The more activities you can check off, the healthier your vagal tone will be. An activated vagal tone translates into:

- Healthy relationships with food and weight: when your SNS and PNS are in balance, you reach satiety when full. You'll be less likely to overeat and gain weight.

- Peaceful demeanor. Anxiety is the result of the SNS being overactive. A balance between the two systems results in less stress.

- Sharp mental functioning. When the SNS takes over, you may develop brain fog. Brain fog can be a very frustrating condition that makes learning difficult.

- Less inflammation. Poor vagal tone allows for chronic inflammation, which is the root of all kinds of chronic diseases.

- Efficient stomach emptying. When the PNS is underactive, food sits in the stomach for long periods. Prolonged food in the stomach results in gas, heartburn, vomiting, bloating.

- Optimism. Depression is associated with differences in parts of the brain, a chemical imbalance, and even an unhealthy gut microbiome. Many of these are side effects of poor vagal tone and can also contribute to depression.

- Ease of swallowing. When the PNS motor neurons aren't working correctly, you may strain your larynx and pharynx.

- Clear, strong voice. The vagus nerve controls most of the larynx muscles so that a healthy vagal tone can mean a clear, loud voice.

- Balance. The pharyngeal branch of the vagus nerve affects the Eustachian tubes, which can affect balance.

- Feeling rested. When the SNS is overactive, sleep can be difficult.

- Normal heart rate. The SNS and PNS balance each other out so that the heart doesn't beat too fast or too slow.

- No heartburn. The PNS is responsible for the release of stomach acids to aid in digestion. An overactive PNS can produce too much and cause heartburn. Likewise, an underactive PNS slows down stomach emptying, which also causes abdominal discomfort.

- Ability to relax. A healthy vagal tone allows one to relax when time allows.

- Joy. An overall sense of health and well-being can cause feelings of pleasure.

Neither of the above lists are complete. It is impossible to list all the advantages of an activated vagus nerve, nor can we list all the ways to stimulate it. Furthermore, we still don't even know all the possibilities of either. Although this is an ancient concept, science is still catching up with the real data to prove it. And we've just seen the tip of the iceberg when it comes to utilizing the vagus nerve for medical intervention.

CHAPTER 9

How Vagal Nerve Stimulation Surgery Helps Prevent Depression

Depression is more than just feelings of sadness that eventually pass. It is a debilitating mental disorder that can ruin one's quality of life. There may be no event or circumstances that caused it, and there may be no end in sight without treatment. It can manifest itself differently in different people, different age groups, and the different genders.

Symptoms of depression in children may involve sadness, anger, irritability, worry, reluctance to go to school, frequent aches and pains, being underweight or overweight, clinginess, and insecurity.

Symptoms of depression in teenagers may include all of the above. Plus, the use of drugs, self-harm, sleeping too much, avoidance of social activities, and loss of interest in things that previously were captivating to them.

Symptoms of depression in adults may present as loss of memory, personality changes, fatigue, loss of interest in sex, physical aches and pains, disinterest in socialization, and suicidal thoughts. Men may be angry while women may be weepier, and the very elderly may simply shut down.

The causes of depression are as mixed as the symptoms. Medical researchers haven't entirely pinned down the root causes. There are some leads, though, as to what may cause some people to be depressed while others in the same situation seem fine. One difference is biological. There may be actual differences in the physical make-up of the brain that makes specific individuals prone to depression. Another difference is brain chemistry. Neurotransmitters in depressed individuals appear to have changed in some capacity as to how they interact with nerves. Brain chemistry alters their function and effect in neuron pathways. Hormones may play a significant role in depression. Hormone changes because of pregnancy, the postpartum period, menopause, and thyroid problems can all trigger depression. And there seems to be some role in inheritance as well. People who have relatives that struggle with depression are more likely to fight bouts of it themselves. Researchers are looking for the genes that may play a part in that.

Treatment for depression can often be successful with medication and talk therapy. The medication works by altering the chemicals in one's brain, and as with any medication, side effects can arise. They can range from jitteriness, dry mouth, diarrhea, and weird dreams to decreased sexual desire, fatigue, blurred vision, and insomnia. Many people try several brands and types of antidepressants until they find one that works well with fewest side effects. Once they find one that is successful, they may remain on it for years, even decades.

Some people, however, may never find an antidepressant that has tolerable side effects. Or if they do manage to tolerate the side effects, the depression isn't alleviated enough to make it worthwhile. Some of these individuals have found relief in surgical vagal nerve stimulation (VNS) therapy. Not everyone can receive this therapy, though. It is reserved for people who have tried four or more antidepressants with little or no success.

VNS therapy was initially approved for epilepsy patients in 1997. It later became recommended for depression patients in 2005. As described in Chapters 6 and 7, the VNS device is a small coiled structure that wraps around the left vagus nerve at the throat level. The right vagus nerve innervates the heart, and stimulation could cause arrhythmia; therefore, doctors usually use the left side. A wire attached to the coil runs under the skin to a small, watch-sized, battery-operated pulse generator placed under the skin on the chest. Its size and concept is much like a pacemaker. The device is surgically implanted on an outpatient basis, and the most significant risk is an infection at the site of the incision. If for any reason, the patient needs to remove the device, that is a simple procedure also.

A few weeks after the surgery, when the incisions have healed, the patient returns to have the electrical pulse generator activated. It can be programmed according to the patient's needs; duration, frequency, and current can be adjusted. Typically, the stimulation begins at a low level, which is gradually increased according to the symptoms. The stimulation will be set to turn on and off in cyclic intervals. A thirty second on and five minutes off range is a typical setting. When the stimulus occurs, there may be a slight tingling or pain in the neck area with hoarseness until the stimulation is over.

Periodic visits will need to be made to the doctor to ensure the device is functioning correctly, the settings are appropriate, the side effects remain tolerable, and symptoms of depression are reducing.

Several side effects can occur with VNS, which include voice changes, hoarseness, throat pain, cough, headaches, shortness of breath, difficulty swallowing, skin tingles, insomnia, and sleep apnea, to name a few. Most patients found these side effects to be tolerable and even lessened with time. Relief from depression doesn't come right away, but within six months, many patients could report a better quality of life. VNS works on depression by stimulating the afferent fibers of the vagus nerve, which carry impulses up to the brain stem where they target regions involved in mood. After many months of stimulation, actual changes in the activity of these regions can be observed.

In a study by Dr. Charles Conway out of Washington University School of Medicine in St. Louis, 600 patients with drug-resistant depression were given VNS therapy. Of that group, only 34% reported a reduction in depression symptoms. Strangely enough, however, they also reported a clinically significant improvement in their quality of life. This improvement in quality of life without a drop in depression symptoms indicates the VNS therapy may be doing something more than just treating depression.

Charles* and Cindy were high school sweethearts. They went to separate colleges but continued to see each other throughout school until they both graduated with their bachelor's degrees. Charles was accepted into a graduate program that would take him across the country, so they decided to get married and go together. Cindy supported them while Charles completed his doctorate in organic chemistry. His internship took them to South Carolina, where they had their first baby. A few years later, Charles landed a prestigious position at a pharmaceutical company. They bought a beautiful house and settled down. They had three more children, and life looked pretty darn good. Charles enjoyed collecting and refurbishing old sports cars, and each new addition was a thrill to him. The kids were all playful and healthy and doing well in school, and his marriage was happy.

Things didn't change overnight. It started very gradually. After a long day at work, he felt too tired to tinker in his extended garage, so the cars he once enjoyed so much sat untouched. The kids' laughter and games that he used to get lured into became slowly more and more of an annoyance. Even Cindy, whom he once felt an almost uncontrollable attraction to, did little to arouse his interest. As time went by, they had less and less romantic involvement despite her attempts to keep the flame alive.

The problems weren't just at home, either, though. Projects at work that once filled him with enthusiasm and ambition were now overwhelming to him. He called in sick frequently, and the company overlooked him for a promotion. Charles just wanted to stay in bed. Sleep was the only relief he could find for the feelings of anger and frustration that had become his most constant companions.

Cindy knew this was not the man she had married. She loved the old Charles, and she wanted him back. She sought the help of their family doctor and eventually convinced Charles to go in for a checkup. Their doctor suggested that Charles go on an antidepressant, and Charles, though skeptical, was so unhappy that he was willing to give it a try. Just as he expected, though, it did very little good and even gave him other problems. They tried another type of antidepressant which had different side effects that were even more unpleasant. They tried another. And another. They tried a combination of medicines, and that led to terrible drug interaction issues.

Charles had just about had it. Suicidal thoughts began to creep into his mind. He was sure that his family would be better off without him. Cindy never gave up, though, and she never stopped loving Charles, even though he could sometimes be challenging. Her faith and the many happy memories they shared, from before Charles got sick, were what carried her through the fear. And every so often, the clouds would part, and Cindy got a glimpse of the brilliant man she fell in love with so long ago.

Moments like that reassured and convinced her that she could find that man again.

Then one morning, while Cindy was making the kids' lunches, she heard of a new treatment for depression in the morning news. It sounded like an answer to her prayers and piqued her interest. Mug of coffee in hand, she abandoned the lunches, sat in front of the TV, poised at the edge of her seat. The procedure, she learned, involved a surgical implant that stimulated the brain's area related to mood. There were very few side effects or risks. Cindy hurriedly finished the lunches, got the kids on the bus, then called her doctor's office. She had to leave a message, but eventually, she got through to him. He had heard of it too but didn't know too much about it. He referred her to a colleague, though, who might be of more help. After several inquiries and a bunny trail of leads, Cindy finally was able to find a clinic that offered the new VNS therapy. She made an appointment for Charles right away.

Charles wasn't nearly as optimistic as Cindy, but he was willing to try. After successfully making it through the screening to see if he was the right candidate for the procedure, they had their appointment for the surgical implant. The morning arrived, and with very mixed feelings between them, they showed up at the clinic where a nurse whisked Charles away. Cindy prayed in the waiting room for this to be the key to open the prison of depression that had kept her old Charles locked away.

The procedure went quickly and smoothly, and a groggy Charles and hopeful Cindy went home that afternoon. A few weeks later, after the incisions had healed, they returned for the follow-up appointment. They were taught how to operate the VNS device, and it was set to a low stimulation. At first, Charles was annoyed by the constant buzzing in his neck every five minutes. Plus, his voice would suddenly get hoarse if he was talking when the vibration occurred.

And to make matters worse, after all that, he didn't even notice any difference in his mood. Once again, he was disappointed. He had several follow-up appointments in the next few months to monitor his symptoms and adjust the settings of his VNS device. Charles didn't hesitate to let the doctor know what a quack job he thought the whole thing was.

Cindy tempered his frustration, though, and reminded him that it would take time.

And she was right. Just as the depression didn't occur all at once, it didn't suddenly disappear either. The subtle changes went almost unnoticed. One morning, about three months after the procedure, Charles woke up and realized that he didn't mind facing all the day's hurdles. Come to think of it; he hadn't minded yesterday either. In fact, last week wasn't so bad. When he got a new assignment at work, he recognized that the old sense of optimism that made him choose his career in the first place. The anxiety and doubt plaguing his projects were becoming nothing more than shadows in a corner that he hoped he'd never be darkened by again. His kids' antics amused him again, and he found himself entering the banter between them. Although they were older now and the types of antics had changed, he found he could still have fun with them, and Charles regretted all the time he had lost with them while they were younger. His garage called to him now too. He had the energy to go tinker on his old cars again after work.

And Cindy? She fell in love again with her Charles. They were like teenagers going out on first dates in the remodeled cars. They'd drive through the countryside, car top down, grinning as the wind blew all those bad memories out of their new life. They had been through hell together, but they made it. Charles reached a point where he didn't even notice the slight vibration in his neck anymore. The scars on his neck and chest didn't bother him either. What he did experience was joy again. He didn't think he'd ever find it, but now each new day became a gift to him.

Charles' story is typical of many patients who have found a new lease on life after finding relief from depression. And although there are very few risks or side effects of the VNS therapy, the noninvasive vagal nerve stimulation (nVNS) treatment may have just as many benefits and even fewer risks or side effects.

Studies from the Universities of Leeds and Glasgow in the United Kingdom have tested this device that fits right into the ear.

The two-week study involved 29 participants who received nVNS therapy every day. In just two weeks of treatment, the researchers found a boost to the parasympathetic nervous system activity while also a reduction in the sympathetic nervous system activity, thus improving the health of the vagal tone. And, some of the study participants also reported a better mood, better sleep, and a better quality of life.

The researchers feel that these findings indicate the beginning of a whole new way to treat depression and a multitude of other health problems.

*Names have been changed to protect the identities of individuals. In some cases, the stories of a few individuals with similar details have been merged into one account.

CHAPTER 10

The Vagus Nerve Stimulation and Reduction of Various Inflammations

Acute Inflammation

Inflammation is the body's defense against injury or invasion. The most familiar form of inflammation is acute inflammation. You've experienced this when you stubbed your toe. It is characterized by five signs: redness, swelling, warmth, pain, and mobility loss if the injury is near a joint. These are all strategies that your immune system is using to protect you. In the proper context, they are all good.

When an injury first occurs, affected cells in the immediate area release chemicals to alert the immune response. Blood rushes to the wound's site, where the capillaries dilate to allow white blood cells through the capillary lining. The infantry unit of white blood cells flood into the offending area.

They will search for invaders to destroy before infection can set in. The redness and swelling are caused by the increase in blood to the area. The heat is caused by the blood also because it quickly came from deeper within your body, where the core temperature is typically warmer than your outer skin. Mobility loss from the excess blood is because there's less room for your joint to move. When the decrease in mobility does occur, though, it makes you less likely to worsen the injury by immobilizing the area, similar to a natural splint. Pain occurs if there are pain receptors in the location of the damage, but it serves a function also. It forces you to protect and treat the area differently, allowing it time and space to heal. If you don't clean the wound properly, unfriendly microorganisms are given access to your body through the skin's opening. A skirmish between the microorganisms and your white blood cells will follow. This battle may result in pus that collects at the site of the action, evidence of the casualties of war.

If the injury is internal, the body's response is similar but perhaps less noticeable. Blood will still rush to the area. The capillaries will again dilate to release the army of white blood cells for their search and destroy mission. This rush of blood causes swelling and perhaps loss of mobility depending on the degree of swelling, pain, and the location. Heat, unless infection has set in, isn't an issue because internal injuries are already at the core body temperature. And pain may or may not occur, depending on whether there are any pain receptors in the area of concern.

Chronic Inflammation

Whether the injury or invasion is internal or external, the acute immune response's effects will last anywhere from a few hours to several days, depending on the severity of the issue. On the other hand, chronic inflammation is a similar response, but its signs may be less noticeable. You may experience fatigue, low-grade fever, random rashes, and dull pain in the chest or abdomen without realizing why. These effects last much longer, though, and can harm the otherwise healthy surrounding tissue over time. You may even reach a point where you are so accustomed to the fatigue, dull pain, and skin irritations that you are barely even aware of them. It becomes your usual mode of operation. This gradual demise is how chronic inflammation can take over your life. Recent studies have implicated chronic inflammation as the leading suspect for a wide range of severe diseases.

There are a few different causes of chronic inflammation. The most obvious is if the acute inflammation is left untreated. A horrifying yet real example of this was in the news a few years ago when a surgeon accidentally left an instrument in his patient's body before sewing it up. The patient experienced unexplainable pain, random bouts of fever, and debilitating fatigue for years before an x-ray for an unrelated exam discovered the offending forceps. Once the forceps were removed, and the lawsuit was underway, the patient had a full recovery.

Another, more frequent, cause of chronic inflammation is an autoimmune disorder. Numerous studies have linked the vagus nerve to this cause of chronic inflammation. Andersson and Tracey in 2012; Tracey in 2016; and Pavlov and Tracey in 2017 have described a response reflex that triggers the vagus nerve to suppress or release the signals to call out the immune response army. However, doctors don't thoroughly understand why, sometimes, the inflammatory reflex goes awry. When this happens, "friendly fire" is the result. The body attacks itself, leading to a plethora of conditions known as chronic disease.

Crohn's disease, rheumatoid arthritis, diabetes, obesity, heart disease, asthma, even Alzheimer's, are just some of the conditions that can be linked to chronic inflammation. During the 2020 Corona Virus Pandemic, the two most significant risk factors for predicting who would suffer the most or die were age and pre-existing chronic diseases. All of those pre-existing diseases are caused by inflammation. Even age, although certainly not caused by inflammation, is amplified by inflammation.

Diet can be a huge factor in controlling inflammation. You should strictly avoid foods such as highly processed carbohydrates, unhealthy fats, sugar, and processed meats that can trigger an immune response. People who have spent their lives eating mostly these types of food will most definitely suffer from some inflammatory condition at some point in their lives. Conversely, olive oil, fatty fish, berries, and green leafy vegetables can all have anti-inflammatory properties. These healthy foods should comprise the majority of your diet. People who eat foods comprised mostly of these items can expect to live in relatively good health well into their old age. Supplements and spices can also help to reduce inflammation. Fish oil supplements and curcumin have been associated with a reduction in inflammation, as well as ginger, garlic, and cayenne pepper.

When dietary changes aren't enough to control the inflammation, you can purchase over the counter nonsteroidal anti-inflammatory drugs (NSAIDs) such as Advil and Aleve. However, long-term use of these drugs can have risks, such as peptic ulcer disease and kidney disease. If diet and NSAIDs don't do the trick, steroids, which you need a pre-scription for, can reduce inflammation and sup-press the immune response. These also have long term risks associated with them. Vision problems, high blood pressure, and osteoporosis are just a few. There are also more immediate side effects, such as weight gain, moodiness, and increased body hair.

Another treatment with very few risks or side effects, however, is now being explored. VNS therapy, previously used to treat epilepsy and depression, is now being studied to inhibit the vagus nerve's immune response.

Infection or injury activates the release of cytokines. Cytokines, a type of protein that signal molecules for the inflammatory response, are produced in the spleen. Still, the vagus nerve inhibits the output in a process called the inflammatory reflex. Studies have found that targeting this reflex with a VNS device in patients with rheumatoid arthritis and Crohn's disease reduces cytokine production.

Rheumatoid Arthritis

Unlike osteoarthritis, rheumatoid arthritis is an immune response that attacks the lining of your joints, causing painful swelling, bone erosion, and joint deformity. It begins in the smaller joints such as fingers and spreads to more substantial joints such as elbows and knees. In most cases, inflammation attacks the joints on both sides of the body. In about

40% of the cases, tissue other than joints can become affected, such as eyes, skin, heart, and lungs. Doctors don't exactly know what triggers this autoimmune disorder. Still, they think that a viral or bacterial response may cause the onset. Traditionally, doctors treat this disease with medication. Not all subjects respond to medication, though.

In a 2019 presentation at the Annual European Congress of Rheumatology, Dr. Mark Genovese, MD, presented the findings of a SetPoint Medical research study on VNS therapy. The study sought to find treatments to alleviate the symptoms of rheumatoid arthritis. He cited an earlier study that involved 17 patients with non-responsive rheumatoid arthritis who had the VNS device surgically implanted. After six weeks of daily 60-second stimulation periods, participants noticed that their symptoms significantly disappeared. Then the researchers turned the VNS device off for two weeks, and the patient's symptoms quickly began to return. Then at eight weeks, the device was turned on again, and symptoms reduced again.

Dr. Genovese then presented the findings of two more recent studies using a newer VNS device model. The more modern device eliminates the need for a chest incision or connecting wire. Instead, they implant the much smaller charge generator in the same location as the coils around the vagus nerve. The patient must plug in a wireless charging apparatus once a week, and the doctor can control the device settings via a smartphone app.

The first recent study he reported had just three participants. They had the new VNS model implanted, and they were given stimulation for one minute per day. These individuals also, very quickly, began to see an improvement in symptoms.

The second recent study involved 11 participants. The researchers divided the participants into three groups. One group received the new VNS model, and the researchers gave them one minute of stimulation once a day. A second group received the new VNS model, and the researchers gave them one minute of stimulation four times a day. The third group received a sham device. Like the previous two studies, the first group noticed a quick and significant improvement in their rheumatoid arthritis symptoms. The second group, interestingly enough, saw no improvement at all. One participant's symptoms even began increasing. There was no change in the symptoms of the sham group.

Although there is still much progress to be made in the blossoming field of bioelectric therapy, these recent studies are very encouraging. Crohn's disease is also in the spotlight as a chronic immunological disorder that may be treatable with VNS therapy.

Crohn's Disease

Crohn's disease, an inflammatory disease that causes inflammation in the colon and latter part of the small intestines, has symptoms which include fatigue, abdominal pain, diarrhea, and weight loss. It can be painful and debilitating and may even lead to life-threatening complications. Doctors don't fully understand what causes the disease, but they think that a viral or bacterial response triggers it. Certain foods and stress can aggravate the symptoms. There is no cure, but there are medications that may reduce the symptoms in some people. But like every treatment plan, there are some people whose disease is resistant to it. In other people, the side effects outweigh the benefits. More than half of the patients with Crohn's disease will need surgery to remove part of the intestines or colon. Even this drastic measure isn't necessarily a cure, though. Eventually, the condition may re-establish itself in the remaining parts of the intestines and colon.

A 2016 study by Bonaz et al. involved seven patients with Crohn's disease. The researchers treated them with cervical VNS. Five of the seven responded positively to the treatment, but two actually worsened. All of them reported voice alteration side effects during stimulation and coughing, pain, and labored breathing. Epilepsy and depression patients reported these same side effects.

In the May 2019 edition of Frontiers in Neuroscience, a study titled, *Anti-inflammatory Effects of Abdominal Vagus Nerve Stimulation on Experimental Intestinal Inflammation*, describes the findings of Payne et al. They induced an inflammatory response in rodents and treated it with VNS. They didn't use cervical VNS, however. The cervical VNS had too many off-target reactions. Besides affecting the pharynx and larynx, heart rate and breathing were also affected. Instead, they wanted to position the VNS closer to the intestines. They devised an apparatus similar to the cervical VNS device, but they implanted it within the abdomen of the rodents. After activating it, they found that nothing other than the intestines were affected. They also found that the device was successful at reducing inflammation in the intestines. They propose that this would be a safe and effective treatment for Crohn's disease in humans.

In a simple search on the topic of VNS therapy and inflammation, many studies will pop up. The frequency of these studies indicates just how hot this topic is right now. With the cost of pharmaceuticals skyrocketing, it's no wonder. If you couple the prices with the side effects and risks of drug interactions, then bioelectric therapy as an alternative treatment becomes a very seductive alternative.

CHAPTER 11

The Strengthening of Vagal Tone and the Reduction of Anxiety

Seth* was thirteen years old when he was diagnosed with a panic disorder. One day, he was in class when suddenly, over the loudspeaker, it was announced that the school would be having an active shooter drill. These drills occur periodically. Although quite stressful initially, most students and teachers in America have gotten used to doing them every month or so. But Seth, although he too has been doing these drills regularly like everyone else, didn't respond like everyone else. While the other 7th graders rolled their eyes and reluctantly got up, looking to their teacher for direction, Seth started to panic. At first, he just paced around, jabbering to no one in particular. Active shooter drills require that everyone remain silent, but Seth couldn't get quiet. When his teacher asked him to stop talking, he ran to her and begged to go to the office to call his mom. Students aren't allowed to go anywhere unattended during a drill. His teacher explained that he could call her in a few minutes when the training was over. Then Seth, a very bright, athletic, popular young man, began to cry. In front of all his classmates. He sobbed that he didn't feel safe and had to get out of the school. Nothing his teacher said to reassure him made any difference. Eventually, the teacher called a school counselor to talk him down. The counselor walked Seth to her office, where he could talk to his mom privately. Long after the drill was over and the lessons had resumed, Seth was finally calming down. His brain understood the entire time that it was just another drill, but he couldn't get his body to understand.

Healthy Anxiety

Anxiety can be quite reasonable, even helpful at times. The queasy feeling you have right before a race is your nervous system getting revved up for action. Adrenaline is coursing through your veins in preparation to help you survive. Your heartbeat increases before you even start to run, and you begin to sweat and feel jittery. Sure, you won't die if you don't win the race, but your body doesn't know that. Your body is merely responding to a stressful situation the best way it knows how. Often some of your best personal record times are run during a race because you've channeled all that 'fight or flight' energy into flight. On a typical practice run, there's nothing to fear, and it takes sheer willpower to knock out a good run. When you're an actor in a play, and you're about to go on stage, you feel like you want to run away or throw up. But instead, you go out there and smile more prominently than you've ever smiled, speak louder than you usually can, and give the performance of your life. It's a beautiful thing, and it's your sympathetic nervous system working on your behalf.

Panic Attacks

But sometimes, anxiety isn't quite as normal, and not quite as healthy. Like Seth, sometimes it's entirely out of place, and no amount of logical reasoning can talk you out of it. Something has triggered a reaction that you are unable to control. Panic attacks are said to be one of the most frightening experiences of one's life. They cause an increased heartbeat, hyperventilation, sweating, and shaking. They can last from ten minutes to an hour or, occasionally, even more. In hindsight, you may not even understand why you had one. You just did, and you couldn't help it. Although many people have had panic attacks and it may have been just a one-time thing. But panic attacks can also be an indicator that there's something more serious going on.

Generalized Anxiety Disorder

Generalized Anxiety Disorder (GAD) is a term used to describe a broad range of anxiety symptoms caused by nonspecific events or situations. People with this disorder may not even know why they are feeling fearful. It is excessive and lasts much longer than a panic attack. GAD can be debilitating if left untreated.

Phobias

Phobias are anxiety disorders that are triggered by specific objects, locations, or events. They are intense, irrational fears from which 19 million people in the United States suffer.

A phobia can be simple or complex, but either way, it is more than just rational fear. People with a simple phobia can get through a typical day with no significant problems. They can accomplish this because they will structure their lives to make sure that they don't run into their trigger. For example, if someone has arachnophobia, intense fear of spiders, they will probably not live in the woods where there are many spiders. They will probably work in a sterile office building where they wouldn't have to face spiders. They would steer away from anything that would be even remotely conducive to harboring spiders. No one would even notice that they have a phobia because they've so successfully learned how to avoid their trigger. A person with a simple phobia would have a day-to-day life that would seem reasonable to anyone who didn't know their personal struggles.

Complex phobias, however, are less discrete. These include social anxiety and agoraphobia. Social anxiety is much more, though than just being shy. People who suffer from it have a crippling fear of humiliation or feeling singled out. Leaving home can be agonizing. Agoraphobia is the paralyzing fear of being unable to escape an open or small space. People with this disorder also can be terrified to leave home. Living a normal life is almost impossible.

Other disorders not listed by The Diagnostic and Statistical Manual of Mental Health Disorders: Fifth Edition (DSM-V) as anxiety disorders; however, anxiety is a large part of them. These include autism, obsessive-compulsive disorder (OCD), and post-traumatic stress disorder (PTSD). In each of these disorders, as well as the ones listed above, the sympathetic nervous system has taken a dominant role in the individual's physiology, causing them to remain in the 'fight or flight' state. This prolonged fight or flight state has profound effects on the brain and the body, leading to a wide range of psychosis, symptoms, and behaviors that are not healthy. These shared symptoms include extreme sensitivity to sounds, weak eye gaze or even gaze aversion, few facial expressions, unusually loud or monotonous speech, and defensive posturing.

Dr. Steven Porges has been a professor and researcher in the study of the vagus nerve and has published more than two hundred peer-reviewed articles. A quick word about the importance of peer review in science. In today's political climate, many people are more likely to listen to politicians' opinions and talk show hosts than to understand the reality of science. But here's how science works; if a scientist publishes a paper in a science journal, it must be peer-reviewed. Peer-review means that other objective scientists have looked over the findings, recreated the experiment or study, and tried to find holes in it. It isn't accepted until those other scientists can confirm the results. So, if someone like Dr. Porges has published over two hundred peer-reviewed papers, it means he has a lot of respect in a community of knowledgeable, objective people who have tried to find his faults. This process of peer-review holds for climate change, gut bacteria, and the coronavirus too. Science is not political. It shouldn't be profit-driven either, though, which is why it is crucial to be skeptical of who is funding the research. Most of these studies included in this book have a disclaimer saying that no funding was associated with their findings.

So, Dr. Porges, a distinguished scientist at the Kinsey Institute at Indiana University and professor of psychiatry at the University of North Carolina, proposed the Polyvagal Theory in 1994 after studying the vagus nerve and publishing scientific papers on it for several decades. This theory describes the vagus nerve as having the commonly accepted pathways described in Chapter 1 of this book, but with one additional unique difference. With convincing evidence, Dr. Porges suggests that the vagus nerve also has two distinct types of fibers in it. The majority of the nerve fibers are unsheathed. In other words, they don't have the protective, fatty layer of insulation called myelin surrounding them. These are the reptilian fibers because they resemble the nerve fibers found in reptiles. Then there are the myelinated fibers that only make up 3% of the vagus nerve. These are the mammalian fibers that are surrounded by fatty insulation. This insulation is essential for the speed and efficiency of the transference of information.

The unmyelinated fibers send information to and from all the organs beneath the diaphragm over

which we have no voluntary control. The myelinated fibers are involved in the organs and tissue
above the diaphragm, which we can sometimes
control. The widely-held belief since the late 1800s
was that we have the two systems mentioned earlier, sympathetic and parasympathetic. These two
systems have been traditionally held responsible for
the balance between our 'fight or flight' reaction
and our 'rest and digest' reaction. Dr. Porges takes
this theory one step further, though. He also suggests that there is a third response that we have no
control over. This third response is an extreme response that only takes over in life and death situations. It is a 'freeze and immobilize' state. TOur
bodies use these hierarchies of response to keep us
alive.

The 'freeze and immobilize' reaction is controlled
by the involuntary, reptilian nerve fibers that communicate with all the organs below the diaphragm.
Just like a reptile will freeze in a panic mode, mammals will also freeze when their body senses a life-
threatening situation. Breathing will stop, the heart
rate will plunge, the legs will turn to "jello," and
the individual may even defecate. Many people

judge victims of rape or abuse because they didn't fight back. Many victims feel shame because they soiled their pants. These are uncontrollable reactions; direct orders from the reptilian nerve that are entirely impossible to control. In extreme cases, the individual will literally die of fear because the heart has stopped.

Anxiety is the body's attempt to keep from entering the 'freeze and immobilize' state. It recognizes that danger is imminent, and it causes movement. Pacing, talking, aggression, increased heart rate, and breathing; these are the classic 'fight or flight' mannerisms. They occur to prevent the shutdown and, as mentioned earlier, can be quite useful and functional. Health problems result, however, when this response remains in gear for too long.

Normal daily functions such as digestion, relaxation, sleep, learning, positive social interactions, play, and reason are all compromised as a result of long term, chronic anxiety. The defensive mechanisms detailed above become the norm. The middle ear, controlled by the vagus nerve, becomes unresponsive, hindering the individual's ability to block background noise and low-frequency sounds. The facial muscles, which are not regulated by the vagus nerve but are closely associated cranial nerves 5 and 7, are no longer expressive. The larynx loses its flexibility, so the voice becomes too loud or monotone. The immune response is compromised. Stomach or bowel inflammation problems arise.

Often, doctors treat chronic anxiety with prescription medications that can have adverse long term effects. Antidepressants, especially selective serotonin reuptake inhibitors (SSRIs), are commonly used to treat many anxiety disorders. Examples of SSRIs include citalopram (Celexa), escitalopram (Lexapro), fluoxetine (Prozac), paroxetine (Paxil), and sertraline (Zoloft). Antihistamines, i.e., hydroxyzine and beta-blockers, i.e., propranolol can be helpful in mild cases of anxiety and performance anxiety, a type of social anxiety disorder. Patients need to take SSRIs every day, whether they feel anxious on that particular day or not. Patients take Antihistamines or beta-blockers only when needed.

Patients who experience panic attacks may need anti-anxiety medication in addition to the antidepressant. The most well-known anti-anxiety drugs are known as benzodiazepines; among them are alprazolam (Xanax), clonazepam (Klonopin), chlordiazepoxide (Librium), diazepam (Valium), and lorazepam (Ativan). Many of these drugs' adverse effects include drowsiness, irritability, dizziness, jitters, nausea, sexual dysfunction, memory and attention problems, dry mouth, weight gain, and physical dependence.

Along with medication, most people who suffer from anxiety are strongly encouraged to seek psychological counseling, psychotherapy, and biofeedback. Biofeedback is a form of therapy where the patient, with the help of a counselor or application, watches brain wave patterns, and learns to control them.

One therapist in Australia who is having unprecedented success in treating all forms of disorders involving anxiety is Holly Bridges. She gives her clients the gift of feeling understood and safe. She teaches them calming techniques that they can do for themselves in any circumstance. Most of all, they learn to trust her, themselves, their body, and eventually, other people.

Holly uses the Polyvagal Theory to work with her clients' built-in survival techniques. She shows them how to listen to their bodies. That is one of Dr. Porges's strongest takeaway points; listen to your body's language. It is trying to protect you. Instead of feeling betrayed by your body, listen to it, be aware of its signals. Anxiety is your body's way of trying to keep you alert in a dangerous situation. Anger is often, especially for men, a more socially acceptable way to express fear. A stomach ache or nausea is another way your body may be trying to tell you that it is afraid. Mindfulness is a meaningful way to slow down and listen to the signals your body is trying to express.

Once Holly has taught her clients to listen to their body, she begins to teach comfort skills to the client. She helps the client realize that their body doesn't need to keep the client in a state of hypervigilance or immobility. The body has to learn to allow the vagal tone to improve and reach a state of healthy equilibrium. And the only way it will be able to get to that point is if it feels safe. Some people, because of early childhood trauma, have never even known how a secure environment feels. They must learn how to find a new, calm normal.

A second take away point, used by Holly Bridges, that Dr. Porges teaches is to find comfort "in the arms of another appropriate mammal." He says this because some people aren't ready yet to trust other people. Still, they can trust a pet and receive social stimulation from that relationship. It doesn't matter if it is a human or a dog or a cat. Dr. Porges says that the most significant way to improve your vagal tone is to have healthy face to face relationships. Nothing can replace eye contact and a prosodic voice and the feeling of being heard and seen.

Infants and children depend on their mothers to meet their needs. Mothers have a natural inclination to speak at a higher frequency, make eye contact, and give hugs; these are all behaviors to which children are naturally drawn. Fathers, though well-intentioned, don't always have those instincts and can't make their voice reach those higher frequencies, leaving some fathers to feel mistakenly rejected by their children. But their children aren't rejecting them, they are simply and naturally fearful of the father's lower frequency voice. Lower frequency sounds such as the roar of a lion, the clash of thunder, the rumble of an approaching stampede are all signals that danger is near. Children feel comfortable through higher frequency sounds. It is inherent. The middle ear is designed to pick up on those sounds of comfort.

There has been an alarming rise in cases of depression and anxiety since the dawn of social media. Instead of fostering personal relationships with neighbors and co-workers and family, we have learned to satisfy that need with posts of pictures, cute stories, likes, and accomplishments. These interactions give us a temporary high, but an overall sense of loneliness. Modern, digital relationships don't meet our ancient, reptilian need to feel safe. As social mammals, we need companionship to believe we are safe indeed. We have to know that someone has our back. We need touch, eye contact, and physical presence.

A third point that Dr. Porges teaches, and that Holly Bridges uses, is breathing. If you take a normal inhale, followed by a long, slow exhale, your heart will naturally slow down. Your reptilian nerve will understand that it is safe. You wouldn't have time, it senses, to breathe that way if you were in danger. Doing breathwork every day will teach your body, over time, that it can relax. Other ways to do this is to play a wind instrument, sing, hum, or do yoga.

Another researcher, Ruairi Robertson, based out of the APC Microbiome Institute in Ireland, studied the effects of the gut biome (bacterial populations living in our intestines) on physical and mental health. In a fascinating study described in a 2015 TEDTalk, *Food for thought: How Your Belly Controls Your Brain*, the researchers replaced the natural gut biome of mice with another type of bacteria. The result of this bacterial transplant caused the mice to lose their natural fear of cats. In fact, he says they became attracted to cats. This intriguing study begs the question, how much of our anxiety is from our brains or our guts? The vagus nerve carries information both ways between the two organs, so the signals of fear can go either way. How often have you felt fear in your gut? Why does anxiety make you nauseous?

Serotonin, the neurotransmitter in our body that makes us feel happy, is primarily produced by the intestines' bacteria. Our brain only makes ten percent. Are we relying on our bacterial populations for our very happiness? Ruairi Robertson and his colleagues have shown that the types of fats we eat affect the types of bacteria that live in our gut. By specifically feeding certain strains of bacteria to mice, we can enhance their memory, change their behavior, and affect their stress. Scientists like Ruairi have developed a list of foods that can stimulate the growth of healthy bacteria, which can reduce stress and anxiety. That list is provided below.

Chapter 8 of this book lists several other techniques that will help strengthen the vagal tone. They are all worth a try, but the most important methods are:

- Accept and appreciate that you have a hierarchy of responses to the environment designed to protect you.

- Listen to those signals of fear with which your body is trying to protect you.

- Reach out to other mammals for comfort and support.

- Practice breathing with long, slow exhales to reassure your body that everything is alright.

- Eat foods that stimulate the growth of healthy bacteria.

Dietary Sources that Stimulate Healthy Microbiome Populations

- Whole Grains
- Apples
- Leeks
- Onions
- Garlic
- Bananas
- Asparagus
- Honey
- Artichokes
- Nuts
- Seeds
- Root Vegetables
- Beans
- Lentils

- Chickpeas
- Green Tea Extracts
- Cocoa Extracts
- Red Wine Extracts

*Names have been changed to protect the identities of individuals. In some cases, the stories of a few individuals with similar details have been merged into one account.

CHAPTER 12

Anxiety and the Role of Vagal Nerve Stimulation in its Reduction

Heart rate variability (HRV) is a scientifically proven means for determining how much stress your body can handle before you begin to have problems from that stress. It's a measure of your resiliency. HRV can predict with 96% accuracy, what your lifespan will be, assuming you don't get unexpectedly hit by a bus or some other unexpected tragedy. Dr. Steven Porges, introduced in the previous chapter, was the first to quantify HRV. The higher the reading, the better your vagal tone and the more excellent your resiliency.

People who suffer from chronic anxiety have a poor vagal tone. Their poor vagal tone is because their rest and relax response isn't able to adjust to the amount of stress the individual's body perceives it to be facing. Therefore, he or she remains in a constant state of fight or flight, which has many long term harmful health risks. Doctors will put patients diagnosed with chronic anxiety or related disorders on an antidepressant and anti-anxiety medication. They are also encouraged to seek counseling as well as therapy. One new form of therapy to treat anxiety is Vagal Nerve Stimulation (VNS).

VNS has been around since the 1930s but wasn't approved for clinical use until 1997 for epilepsy. Its use in the treatment of epilepsy and depression can be read in Chapters 6 and 9, respectively. If you'd like to review procedures, side effects, and benefits, they are in Chapter 7. Using VNS to treat stress isn't an especially profound concept, given that stimulating the vagus nerve is known to produce calming effects, and anxiety is a lack of calm. The profound aspect of VNS therapy on stress is the recent improvements that researchers are now making on the product. Besides the slick new non-invasive (nVNS) designs, the products are available for consumers to purchase, if they'd like, for around $300 - $400.

Neuvana produces an nVNS device, called Xen, that has shown decided improvements in people's mood and overall sense of well-being. It is a round, flat stimulation generator about the size of a makeup compact that fits into your pocket. It then plugs into your cell phone, where an app allows you to adjust the settings. It also can connect with Spotify or any other music stream of your choice. It has normal-looking earbuds that then play the music while also providing the VNS therapy through the auricular branch of your vagus nerve. The Xen by Neuvana is such a forward-thinking device that it won the iPhone Consumer Electronics Show Best of 2020 Award.

Another new nVNS device is called the Sensate Pebble. It is a necklace with a teardrop-shaped device that fits in the palm of your hand. You lay down with the instrument resting on your chest for just ten minutes per day. The company even provides a satin seed pillow for laying over your eyes to assist with relaxation. You can wear it like a big necklace as you go about your daily activities as well. The Sensate Pebble produces a sound that you can't hear and vibrations that you can feel on your sternum. The noise and the vibrations combine to stimulate the vagus nerve. The company boasts an 86% improvement in heart rate variability after just six weeks of daily use.

Matthew Hatson gives a comparison of the two products on YouTube. He tried them each individually for a month. His opinion is that the Sensate Pebble is a better choice for someone new to understanding brain/body interactions through the vagus nerve. Someone who isn't very aware of the signals the body is giving to slow down and focus on calming techniques may need the set schedule suggested. This suggestion is because the ten minutes per day of laying down with the device on your chest is a great way to learn calming techniques and breathing practices.

Someone who already uses many of the vagus nerve activation tricks and is aware of their breathing to reset the system may be happier with the Neuvana Xen. It is a much more discrete product, for one thing, as it looks as if you're just wearing earbuds. Second, according to Matthew Hatson, it gives a more noticeable calming effect, a more substantial boost to your vagal tone, and better HRV in the long run.

There are becoming more of these products on the market as this new branch of therapy unfolds and offers help for an ever-growing list of disorders. These are two of the most popular. What are some advantages of using this therapy over meditation and yoga and other previously discussed techniques? The main one is consistency because it can be difficult to do yoga or meditation every day. Plus, not everyone has the patience and discipline to do either practice. nVNS offers an easy way to keep your vagal tone healthy daily, no matter how busy your schedule. Brain scans of people using devices like these are comparable with those who have been practicing meditation techniques for ten years.

Janice* had been struggling with anxiety for years. Her anxiousness prevented her from doing many of the activities for which she envied other people. Janice had stomach ulcers on top of that, which only made her anxiety worse. She was on medication but worried about the long-term risks involved. Janice wanted to do meditation because of the benefits it offered. Still, she just couldn't train her brain to focus on "nothing" for more than a few seconds. After several failed attempts at several forms of meditation, she quit trying. When she heard about the new nVNS devices on the market, she became intrigued. Yes, $400 was a lot to pay for something that may or may not work, but what if it did work? She'd spent three times that to go to her chiropractor regularly. Isn't mental health just as important, if not more important, than physical health? Can there even be physical health without mental health?

Janice finally decided to go for it. She immediately felt different after her first day. She felt happier and less stressed. Encouraged, she also bought an HRV monitor to track her progress. Each day felt better and better, and the incremental climbing of her HRV provided additional support. Within a year, she had the HRV of someone who had been practicing yoga and meditation for ten years. The nVNS was one app Janice never regretted.

*Names have been changed to protect the identities of individuals. In some cases, the stories of a few individuals with similar details have been merged into one account.

CHAPTER 13

The Vagus Nerve and Trauma

Angie* was at home one Sunday afternoon, going through the week's menu and grocery list when she realized a helicopter had been circling over her home for a little while. At first, she hadn't even noticed it, but the steady drone of the blades made its way to her nerves, and all at once she realized she was annoyed. Angie lived in a neighborhood where there was a large elderly population, though. Hence, she figured it was a silver alert. She returned to her planning, and eventually, the helicopter moved on.

Angie didn't think about the distraction again until she left her home to go to the grocery store. As she left her secluded home, she saw that the road was lined with emergency vehicles, one of which was a forensics unit. She texted her neighbor, Debbie, to see if she knew anything. Debbie didn't respond, but that wasn't unusual. Debbie had a teenage son,

Jonathon, and was often busy with sporting events. Angie usually left a message, knowing Debbie would get back to her as soon as she could.

Angie did her grocery shopping and ran a few more errands before returning home. Debbie still hadn't returned the phone call, and Angie was beginning to feel nervous. They had grown up together, both returning to their childhood homes after their parents, also good friends, decided to downsize and move to a retirement village. Now they were both mothers and raising their children in the same woods they had grown up in together. Debbie had been having some issues with her son, though. Angie suspected drugs were involved because her daughter shared rumors from school about Jonathon with her. But Angie didn't feel Debbie was ready to have that conversation yet. It was beginning to come between them. Debbie wouldn't, or couldn't, face the reality of her son's erratic behavior.

By the time Angie went to bed that night, Debbie still hadn't returned the call. A growing feeling of anxiety was beginning to manifest itself in Angie.

Early the next morning, an agent from the Department of Child Services rang Angie's doorbell, and with the agent was Jonathon. Not yet a legal adult, Jonathan, who was 17, explained that his mother had been mysteriously stabbed to death while taking a nap yesterday afternoon. The helicopter yesterday had been searching the woods for the murderer. Jonathon had been questioned by the police all night and needed a place to stay temporarily. Immediately, Angie felt the blood rush out of her head, and her legs go to jello. She fell against the front door for support as she processed the devastating news.

The agent explained that it would only be for a few days until they could find a more permanent situation. When she regained control of her emotions from the news of her life-long friend, Angie struggled with the decision. A gut feeling told her that Jonathon was the knife-wielding murderer, but what if she was wrong? What if he was just a kid, reeling from the loss of his mother. Angie felt she had no choice. She took him in but spent the entire week in a constant state of hyper-alert, fearing for her own life and the lives of her adult children who were visiting. Was there a murderer wandering around her woods, waiting for an opportunity to attack his next victim? Or was the murderer in her guest bedroom waiting for her to fall asleep?

The longest week of Angie's life crawled by as she waited for DCF to place Jonathon in a foster home. It was an awkward week of intensely mixed feelings: grief, fear, suspicion, sympathy, anger, guilt. Everything came to a halt, and normal life couldn't resume until some resolution occurred. To stay busy, Angie spent most of her time cooking for her family and guest. Angie had to have hushed phone conversations with concerned family and friends outside, away from Jonathon's hearing.

Angie stayed in contact with the police as they continued their investigation. They couldn't tell her much, other than that Jonathon was a person of interest. Two weeks after he showed up on her doorstep, DCF took Jonathan to a foster home. A few months later, he finally confessed to having killed his mom in a drug-induced rage. Angie had nightmares for months and found herself crying about insignificant things like burnt toast, rather than the violent loss of her oldest friend. Her pastor explained that she was suffering from acute indirect trauma and gave her some exercises to relieve the stress, including prayer and writing in a journal. If she didn't feel better soon, she knew she would need to see a doctor.

Trauma

The word "trauma" can be used in two senses, although they are similar. Physically, trauma means an injury that needs to heal. Psychologically, it means the same thing. Whether it's physical, as in Debbie's case that killed her, or psychological, as in Angie's case that temporarily crippled her, something violent has happened. If victims don't take precautions to address the trauma, it could lead to worse problems or even death. The vagus nerve plays a part in both forms of the word.

Psychological Trauma

First, though, before we look at the vagus nerve, psychological trauma can be further divided into several categories. There is acute trauma, where a one-time incident has left emotional scars on an individual. There is chronic trauma, where an individual has been exposed to prolonged physical or emotional abuse. There is complex trauma, which occurs when an individual has been exposed to different personal and invasive events that have affected their overall well-being. Insidious trauma, another form, isn't necessarily directed at you, but rather, at a group with which you identify. Racism, sexism, gangs, are examples of situations that can cause insidious trauma. There is also direct or indirect trauma. Direct trauma happens to you; indirect trauma affects you because it happens to someone or something you care about. Organizational trauma affects people who belong to an organization where something traumatic occurs. Secondary traumatic stress affects health care workers who care for victims of an event. No matter what type of psychological trauma an individual may face, just like physical trauma, further problems can result if the victim doesn't take care of the issue.

Acute Trauma

Angie was an otherwise healthy, well-adjusted adult when the violent murder of her friend occurred. It was a single event that disrupted her entire sense of world order. Acute trauma occurs when a one-time event completely and violently rattles the world of an individual. Acute trauma can be direct or indirect trauma, depending on if the incident happened directly to you or to someone or something about which you care. The impetus can be a wide range of single events such as murder, rape, 9/11, an earthquake, or a car accident. The symptoms involve feelings of shock or disassociation. They can cause recurring nightmares or thoughts, continually returning to the event. If left unresolved, this situation can lead to acute stress disorder (ASD), which could further lead to post-traumatic stress disorder (PTSD). We will address these in Chapter 15.

Chronic Trauma

On the other hand, chronic trauma is an on-going situation that can result in multiple traumatic episodes lasting for years. Veterans, victims of child abuse, slaves in the horrific sex trafficking underworld, battered spouses; these are all scenarios that can last for years, even decades. Child sex slaves and victims of domestic child abuse or neglect may not even know that there is an alternative to feeling fearful. They don't even know what they don't know; that hurt isn't normal. And this is especially tragic because their young minds are still developing. Severe trauma can alter the development of their brain, leaving life long physical and psychological scars. More will be discussed on the impact of trauma on brain development in the next chapter.

A study in the mid-90s done by the Center for Disease Control (CDC) surveyed seventeen thousand adults who had survived traumatic childhood events. This demographic was made up of 70% college-educated, Caucasians. The CDC and the United States Substance Abuse and Mental Health Services Administration came up with an official list of adverse childhood experiences (ACEs). These are:

- Physical abuse

- Sexual abuse
- Emotional abuse
- Physical neglect
- Emotional neglect
- Family members treated violently
- Substance misuse within the household
- Parental separation or divorce
- Incarcerated household member

These stressful or traumatic events can be direct or indirect. They may also include household dysfunction, such as witnessing any of the above. The people who are aware of abuse or neglect, but are powerless to stop it, can feel almost as victimized as the person on the receiving end of the violation.

The prolonged exposure to or experience of these events is strongly related to a wide range of health problems throughout a person's lifespan. Being able to check off three or more of these events makes you susceptible to the mental and physical health struggles of PTSD. Over half of all Americans report surviving at least one of the above situations. One in eight Americans can check off four or more, which can mean a twenty-year difference in life expectancy.

Dr. Robert Block is the former President of the Academy of Pediatrics. He said, "Adverse childhood experiences are the single greatest unaddressed public health threat facing our nation today." ACEs are a threat because if you can check off having experienced four or more of these ACEs, you are more than two times more likely to have high blood pressure as an adult. You're also more than two times more likely to come down with hepatitis. You're more than four times more likely to be depressed and TWELVE times more likely to attempt or consider attempting suicide. Furthermore, if you can check off seven or more ACEs, you're three times more likely to be diagnosed with lung cancer. You're also three and a half times more likely to get the number one killer in the United States, chronic heart disease.

Six million Americans have active PTSD symptoms, and millions more have partial PTSD symptoms.

Complex Trauma

We could easily use the term complex trauma to describe 2020. Regardless of nationality, residents of Earth have experienced a pandemic which has left millions of people dead, grieving, very ill, out of work, or in some cases, overworked. As a result of the pandemic, the quarantine has left many of those same people with no income or trapped in an abusive situation at home. Caregivers are in impossible situations because they may not want to return to their homes at the risk of exposing their families to COVID. The racial riots and demonstrations resulting from the death of an unarmed black man, George Floyd, in the custody of police have rocked the world as well. Many of the same people who have suffered from illness, grief, and economic stress are now facing racial injustice issues. They may have been involved in violent clashes that have left them or a loved one injured, in jail, or with their business shattered. And yet, despite these unprecedented times, no one is exempt from the ordinary life tragedies that continue to plague humanity. These tragedies include refugees who are still homeless and car accidents that are still happening.

It encompasses the trauma of people who are diagnosed with terminal cancer and marriages that are still ending. Crime continues, hurricanes season approaches, wildfires rage. The harsh reality of everyday life marches on. There is no other way to explain all these events happening at once but very complex. 2020 is exceptionally complicated complex-trauma.

Insidious Trauma

On top of all the complex trauma outlined above, in a very literal sense, the Black American community has suffered from insidious trauma. Studies of epigenesis find that chronic trauma affects an individual's DNA, how it is read and transcribed, and which genes get turned on or off. Trauma affects the genes of the victim, but also those genetic alterations are then passed down to subsequent generations. The sorrow and suffering afflicted on their enslaved forefathers have genetically affected today's Black Americans, resulting in many of the symptoms of stress and trauma. Deeper still, they may feel hopeless in a system that perpetuates generational poverty. They are the victims of a power struggle for which they didn't ask. Other victims of insidious trauma are refugees. For political, environmental, or religious reasons, they have lost their homes. Now they are forced to live in squalid, crowded, disease-ridden camps. The DNA of these people may be altering now, affecting generations to come.

Organizational Trauma

As companies collapse into bankruptcy this year from a loss of income, civil unrest, or property damage, entire communities of people who once thought of themselves as a team are finding themselves lost. Organizational trauma leaves them jobless and worried about their future. Some may define their identity based on their position in the company and the relationships they built within those walls. In other situations, a beloved co-worker may die unexpectedly, leaving the entire organization crippled, emotionally, and functionally.

Secondary Trauma

Finally, as mentioned above, healthcare workers have faced unimaginable horrors. They helplessly watched one patient after another suffer and die alone from Covid-19. There have been several recent news stories of them taking their own lives due to the weight of being asked to help too many people, with too few resources, and no real plan of healing. They've endured the risk of their own lives and those of their loved ones. They've lost colleagues who have succumb to the infection or suicide. They have fought the unorganized approach to battle the odds. And they have struggled with sheer exhaustion. One nurse describes a night when she finished her shift, exhausted and drained, leaving the care of her twenty-five patients in the hands of the next shift. When she returned the following day, ten of the twenty-five were dead. She and the rest of the health care workers in the hardest-hit areas have been experiencing secondary trauma.

The Vagus Nerve's Role in Trauma

So how does trauma relate to the vagus nerve? First off, let's go back to physical trauma. Studies have shown that the vagus nerve is integral to the immune response. We call it the immune response reflex because it happens instantly and involuntarily, just like any other reflex. Once chemicals from damaged cells are detected, the vagus nerve relays that information to the brain. Then the brain sends instructions back for the spleen to release other chemicals. This response is detailed more in Chapter 10. What's interesting to note here is what we can do with this information. A study in 2010 by Czura et al., *Vagus Nerve Stimulation Regulates Hemostasis in Swine,* indicated that a 40% reduction in bleeding occurred after they administered VNS to injured swine. They suggested that this discovery could be used to pre-treat patients before an operation to prevent excessive bleeding. This discovery could make operations less complicated and speed up healing.

Now, on to psychological trauma. The polyvagal theory, proposed by Dr. Steven Porges, was introduced in the previous chapter. It contends that the vagus nerve has an ancient, reptilian component to its fibers. This unmyelinated pathway is responsible for the third type of reaction to environmental conditions. Typically we think of just two reactions to environmental conditions. We know the rest and digest response, which relaxes us when there is no danger, and the fight or flight response prepares us for action when there is danger.

The third response, freeze and immobilize, shut us down completely when the danger is too overwhelming. It is an overreaction of the vagus nerve, but it has its place. It is protective to prevent suffering. When the danger is life-threatening or too emotionally painful to bear, the vagus nerve simply removes you from the situation. Angie began to enter this response when she found out about Debbie's murder. Angie's knees buckled, her head began to swim, and she had to fall into the door for support. Hopefully, Debbie went completely into this response before she died. If so, she wouldn't have suffered too much physically and emotionally, knowing that it was her son who was murdering her. Rape and abuse victims may wonder why they didn't fight, but the reality is that they couldn't. They were rendered motionless by their bodies.

*Names have been changed to protect the identities of individuals. In some cases, the stories of a few individuals with similar details have been merged into one account

CHAPTER 14

Signs and Symptoms of Trauma and Its Impact on the Brain

In the previous chapter, both physical and psychological trauma were addressed, and the vagus nerve's role in each was explored. In describing the symptoms of trauma, the physical can shed light on the psychological. What happens to a bone if it breaks, and we don't give it the proper treatment to heal? It may heal on its own incorrectly and result in a deformed limb. Pain may cause avoidance of the use of that limb. Infection and inflammation may set in to produce even more symptoms. The same is true with psychological trauma. If it isn't addressed correctly, misshapen or misappropriate behaviors may be activated. Avoidance of triggers may occur, and chronic inflammation may set in, resulting in even more symptoms.

Also, in Chapter 13, different forms of trauma were described and classified, and they all share a common thread. That common thread is fear, reaction to the fear, and the support we receive through the fear. Fear is the second most powerful force through which we must navigate. It is what causes us to shift between the three polyvagal responses. If we feel no fear, we can happily exist and function in the rest and digest state. If we feel fear, we will either fight, flee, or freeze. A traumatic experience forces us into one of those reactions to fear. If we have a healthy vagal tone with plenty of support and awareness, we will quickly return to the rest and digest state when the trauma has passed. However, if that trauma is prolonged or we don't have support or aren't able to process it, healing and recovery can't begin. And just like a broken bone, other complications start to arise.

As humans, we have a highly developed ability to absorb and process a constant flow of sensory input. From the moment our brain is advanced enough, we start filing the new sights, sounds, tastes, feelings, and smells into "safe" and "unsafe" filing cabinets in our minds. Also, the more any sensory experience fits within our expectations, the less memorable it is. People who find themselves in a traumatic circumstance are experiencing something that is usually very unexpected and categorically unsafe. How old they are when the trauma occurs, how long it lasts, and how they recover is the difference between having post-traumatic stress or post-traumatic growth.

Symptoms and Behaviors Associated With Trauma

Post-traumatic stress can have many symptoms. Frequent flashbacks, nightmares, night sweats, insomnia, unexplained anxiety, depression, panic attacks, control issues, difficulty concentrating, resistance to positive change, and avoidance issues can be indicators that a person needs to resolve their traumatic experience. These symptoms mean that the individual is still in some form of the fight, flight, or freeze response, which inhibits the rest and digest processes needed for health. This repression of rest and digest leads to so many of the physical disorders and behaviors that can be associated with post-traumatic stress.

At least nine learned behaviors appear to be "personality traits" of someone with post-traumatic stress disorder (PTSD). They include difficulty concentrating and gaps in memory, a strong need to be in control of anything that affects them, and an inability to ask for genuine help. They may ask for superficial demonstrations of "help," but that is just them asserting control, in their minds, over someone. Actual help would mean they admit a real problem, which they strictly avoid, and any resignation to positive change. In their attempts to maintain the facade of being in control, perfectionism and fear of failure can be quite common. Oddly enough, at the same time, fear of success and low self-esteem are underlying tigers hidden in the grass. These inner struggles and worries may cause them to physically or emotionally lash out, hurting themselves and others. If any of this sounds like narcissistic tendencies, there are some commonalities. Early childhood abuse or neglect, whether mild or severe, can create a narcissistic individual with PTSD. The need to be accepted and loved caused many of the learned behaviors, which, at the time, may have served them well. Furthermore, in today's culture, many of those tendencies are applauded, rather than squelched, leading to even more pronounced expressions of those acquired traits.

Physical Complications Associated With Trauma

Fear suppresses the relaxation response. People may fear a loss of control. They may fear failure, or people not perceiving them as perfect. They may fear the underlying traumatic circumstances that launched the hyper-vigilant behaviors are all culprits of suppressing the relaxation response. When the body's natural state of equilibrium is altered because it is hyper-alert, the vagus nerve isn't able to function optimally. This hyper-alert state caused by fear, as we've covered throughout this book, affects heart rate, breathing, blood pressure, digestion, toxin elimination, and the immune response. Therefore, people who have PTSD often suffer from chronic disease. Chronic disease includes heart attacks, high blood pressure, strokes, chronic fatigue, digestion problems including constipation, diarrhea, heartburn, ulcers, and inflammatory problems such as obesity, diabetes, irritable bowel syndrome, and many more.

As mentioned previously, one of the vagus nerve's primary roles is to regulate the inflammatory reflex. Without this response, inflammation runs rampant in the body. As pointed out in Chapter 10, unchecked inflammation is responsible for almost every chronic disease known to man. And most of these diseases are especially familiar to trauma victims. Western medicine all too often treats each of these maladies individually with medications which merely act as a bandaid. The goal needs to be getting the body back into the relaxation response so that the vagus nerve can properly regulate all the visceral organs. The relaxation response can't happen, though, if there are unresolved fears, or psychological injuries, from the trauma.

Back to our brain's filing system, as we progress through life, our two filing cabinets get more and more filled with "safe" and "not safe" folders. When we experience a traumatic event, there can be sensory experiences that get put into the "unsafe" filing cabinet which, under normal circumstances, wouldn't be in the "unsafe" category:

Jim*, only 19 and new to the army, was sleeping in a tent in Vietnam in 1974 with two close buddies when he awoke to the sound of rain. At first, it was just a soft pitter-patter, but eventually, it escalated into a torrential downpour. The storm was so loud that he didn't hear the approach of an airplane. The airplane dropped a bomb which exploded in very close proximity to his tent. He passed out. When he woke up, he was covered in blood and body parts; one friend was dead, and the other had lost both legs. Jim was injured, but he recovered physically. He returned to battle to experienced many other unfathomable traumatic events and the loss of too many close friends. Fortunately, the war didn't last much longer, and Jim returned home to Seattle.

When Jim returned home, his head knew he was back and safe. Still, his nervous system remained on hypervigilance from being in that mode for so long and not resolving the experiences he had. Jim suffered from nightmares and irritable bowels. After losing so many loved ones, he was very reluctant to respond to any close relationships. The most challenging problem he faced, however, was his reaction to the sound of rain. It triggered an irrational fear of being that young, vulnerable, brand new soldier about to get attacked, lose his best friends, and lose his innocence. It caused anxiety, which manifested as restlessness, sweating, panic attacks, anger, and sometimes violence. When the rain stopped, it left him shaky and exhausted with the need to smoke and drink strong alcohol. He'd pass out after numbing his senses, only to find himself in a similar situation in a nightmare. He so profoundly hated rain that he moved to Arizona, where he could avoid it as much as possible. But one can't always control everything, and that fear never wholly left the hidden recesses of his mind.

Once Jim settled down in Arizona, he found a support group and was able to resolve many issues. He was even able to form reasonably healthy relationships, hold down a respectable job, have a family, and lead a healthy life as long as it didn't rain. Jim just couldn't shake the fear that rain caused. He managed it so most people wouldn't even notice, but he knew it was there. He knew how hard he was working to appear normal each time he heard the first few drops of the occasional storm. Fortunately, it didn't often rain, nor did it rain for very long where he lived, and he had no desire to travel to parts of the world that had more rain. Even his wife didn't know how distressing the rain was to him.

When they retired, and the children were grown, his wife desperately wanted to see the world. Jim knew he wouldn't be able to handle his fear of the rain, coupled with the uncertainty of unfamiliar surroundings. Without explaining, he simply refused. This stubborn silence led to fights and frustration between his wife and him. It drove a wedge between them because his wife didn't understand why he was such "an old stick in the mud." After enough fighting, during a moment of intimate conversation, Jim finally confessed his real reason for not wanting to travel. As his wife reflected over their years together, things began to make more sense. Normally very stable and steady, Jim's infrequent bouts of irritability and withdrawal almost always coincided with bad weather.

Jim always said his wife was very stubborn, and this situation was no different. Although she was now sympathetic to his problem, she wasn't ready to have if affect her plans for the future. She was determined to get help for them, which brought them to virtual reality exposure therapy (VRET).

Virtual Reality Exposure Therapy

One of the more successful treatments for people with post-traumatic stress is prolonged exposure therapy. It exposes the victim to the very thing they fear in a safe and gentle environment, starting briefly and slowly while progressing to longer, more intense exposure.

Virtual reality has gained usefulness as a tool for prolonged exposure therapy. While once too expensive and unrealistic, technological maturity has made it now more reasonable, adaptive, and realistic. As a result of VRET, Jim grew to be able to allow himself to be surrounded by simulated rain. He was able to vary the intensity of the storm, the shower's location, and the duration of the rain. It took time, talk therapy, support, patience, and tenacity, but slowly Jim was able to face a real storm in any situation, calmly and confidently. And his wife achieved her dream to travel extensively with her husband.

Jim was one of the lucky ones, though. Many people with PTSD aren't always able to subject themselves to stillness and calm. They may not even know what triggers their symptoms. They find the quiet to be stressful because it allows their fears to close in around them. So they fight it. They stay busy. They talk. They fidget. They get angry. They remain restless. ...And it wreaks havoc on their physical health and brain physiology.

Changes in the Brain

The parts of the brain affected by trauma are primarily the nucleus accumbens, the amygdala, the hippocampus, and the prefrontal cortex. The nucleus accumbens is a central player in reward and pleasure. It helps in the discipline of delayed gratification. The amygdala, which isn't much bigger than an almond, is located on both sides of the cerebral hemispheres. It is responsible for taking in sensory signals, controlling motivational behaviors, and experiencing emotions. It is also involved in activating the adrenal gland to release the stress hormones, adrenaline, and cortisol. The hippocampus is where memory formation occurs, and it is located deep in the temporal lobe. It also is essential in regulating emotional response. The prefrontal cortex is where we make choices, and where we reason. It is part of the brain's frontal lobe and helps determine personality and social behavior.

Depending on when the trauma occurred while the brain was developing, there can be permanent physiological differences between the brains of trauma survivors and healthy individuals'. A 2006 study by Dr. David Bremner, *Traumatic Stress: Effects on the Brain,* found that an overactive amygdala and a failure of the medial prefrontal cortex to extinguish or shut off, the amygdala, when the immediate threat is no longer an issue was evident in people living with PTSD versus healthy individuals. Trauma inhibits the prefrontal cortex, causes measurable differences in the size of the hippocampus, and causes the amygdala to be hyperactive. Other studies have demonstrated that if help isn't received soon after the trauma, those differences could be permanent. This damage may result in memory loss, impulse control, inappropriate fear reactions, and future stress responses. The more time elapsed after a traumatic event has occurred, the fewer chances there are for therapeutic healing.

*Names have been changed to protect the identities of individuals. In some cases, the stories of a few individuals with similar details have been merged into one account.

CHAPTER 15

Treatment of Post-Traumatic Stress Disorder Through Vagal Nerve Stimulation

Vagal nerve stimulation (VNS) has been thoroughly described in Chapter 6 concerning the treatment of epilepsy, and Chapter 9 about depression. Chapter 10 explored its effect on inflammation, and Chapter 12 described its influences anxiety. It is clear that in each instance, its success as an effective treatment is in its proven ability to stimulate the vagus nerve. This stimulation gives the parasympathetic nervous system a boost, improving the overall health of the vagal tone. And in each of those maladies, the primary cause of the symptoms seems to be an overactive sympathetic nervous system. Post-traumatic stress disorder (PTSD) is no different.

If you are in a life and death situation during an emergency, your sympathetic nervous system's fight or flight response is possibly going to save your life. There have been many stories of people accomplishing superheroic feats that they, even, can't believe. One commonly told story is of a person lifting an entire vehicle off someone trapped underneath. In another story, the Bible speaks of David as a young boy, tending his father's sheep, catching bears and lions by the jaw, and clubbing them to death as they tried to steal a lamb. The fight or flight response floods the body with adrenaline, and superhuman strength becomes possible. This sympathetic response is entirely appropriate in emergency moments like these.

But, thankfully, we don't experience too many moments like these, so most of the time, we should be chilling in our rest and digest phase. Most of the time, we should be relaxed and social and healthy and happy. But people who have been through any form of trauma, as was revealed in the previous two chapters, may not be able to return to that phase. Their fear response may be permanently on, waiting for the next nonexistent lion or bear. Their par-asympathetic nervous system needs a boost to over-ride the sympathetic nervous system. Only two drugs (sertraline and paroxetine) are approved by the US FDA to treat PTSD. These medications re-duce symptom severity but may not produce a com-plete remission of symptoms. All the medicine or therapy in the world won't help if you don't con-vince the body that it's safe.

The first, most obvious way to convince the body that it's safe is to remove it from the danger. Re-moval from danger may mean distancing yourself from people who are toxic or moving to a safer neighborhood or finding a less stressful job. The next way to convince the body that it's safe is to allow it to feel the support of a tribe. We have de-veloped, over the eons, as social animals. Even the most extreme introvert needs some form of social interaction for the body to feel safe. As Dr. Steven Porges pointed out, "find safety in the arms of an-other appropriate mammal." It doesn't have to be human interaction, but it does have to be emotion-ally close and face-to-face support. Sometimes, for whatever reason, you can't remove yourself from the dangerous situation. Hopefully, though, you can find comfort from other people or animals in that situation with you. There have even been stories of prisoners of war, trapped in solitary confinement, who found comfort in the company of the rats and cockroaches that shared their cell.

Once you meet those two criteria as much as possible, the other forms of vagus nerve activation will be much more effective. Breathwork, which has already been detailed and will be explored again in the next chapter, is a most useful and effortless, inexpensive way to boost vagal tone. Breathwork can be expedited further with the help of an HRV biofeedback device. Biofeedback allows you to see, in real-time, how your breathing is helping your HRV. It involves wearing a clip on your ear that will sync with an app on your phone. It instructs you how to breathe and monitors the effect it's having on your HRV. With consistent use, you can achieve permanent improvements —more on this in Chapter 17.

Another successful device is the VNS device. Although initially developed and approved in 1997 for treatment-resistant epileptic patients, it was observed that the device seemed to improve users' general mood. It then, in 2005, became approved for treatment-resistant depression. In 2015, it was cleared to treat obesity. Since then, the medical research community has embraced the many possibilities the VNS device has to offer. Because it improves vagal tone, the possibilities are limitless. And because PTSD has so many comorbidities, VNS is a very appealing solution. Although still in the research stage, studies have found VNS to be effective in rats if paired with exposure therapy. VNS seems to reduce the fight or flight impulse when the recipient is exposed to the fear-inducing object, thus allowing the brain more plasticity for relearning sensations concerning that object.

In Psychology Today, May 23, 2014, *How Does the Vagus Nerve Convey Gut Instincts to the brain?*, another study done on rats severed the afferent vagal fibers from the stomach to the brain. This procedure prevented the rats from unlearning fear in a conditioned response to sound. However, they were less afraid of things they would generally be fearful of, such as bright lights and open spaces.

In other words, without the afferent vagal fibers, the rats' gut instincts were less sharp in naturally dangerous situations. At the same time, learned fears of otherwise harmless stimuli were more pronounced. These findings support the hypothesis that vagal nerve stimulation could be beneficial to people living with PTSD.

A few, minimal, studies in humans have found positive results on PTSD symptoms with VNS alone. Further research needs to be done on the pairing of VNS with exposure therapy on humans. Although it has shown to be successful in rats, researchers have not determined whether VNS will hasten or impair the human brain's plasticity during exposure therapy.

With the help of the nVNS device, we can reduce anxiety, which is vital since stress is the umbrella under which PTSD resides. With anxiety reduced, depression and suicidal thoughts can be erased as well as substance abuse. Furthermore, inflammation can be brought under control. Without inflammation, we can eliminate high blood pressure, heart disease, lung cancer, irritable bowel syndrome, dementia, diabetes, and asthma.

CHAPTER 16

Yoga and the Vagus Nerve

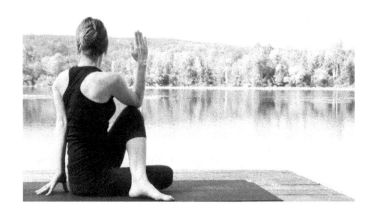

History of Yoga

We can find evidence of yoga as early as 2300 BCE in the Harappan civilization, the earliest known Indian subcontinent's urban culture. There, lotus positioned drawings of Shiva, a Hindu god, were found. But yoga didn't become widely popular in India until Maharishi Patanjali penned the Yoga

Sutra in 300 BCE. We actually know very little about Patanjali other than that he was born in Benares, India, and that yogis consider him to be the Father of Yoga. His document listed 195 rules for integrating yoga into daily living. We can divide the Yoga Sutras into eight categories of regulations.

- Yama – Five principles of ethics: The five Yamas ask practitioners to avoid violence, lying, stealing, wasting energy, and possessiveness.

- Niyama – Five principles of conduct & discipline: The five Niyamas ask us to embrace cleanliness and contentment, purify ourselves through heat, study and observe our habits continually, and surrender to something greater than ourselves.

- Asana – Physical practice of yoga: These physical movements are the main focus of Westernized yoga.

- Pranayama – Breath regulation: Practitioners of yoga usually include this into many popular yoga disciplines.

- Pratyahara – Sensory withdrawal: Anything that takes your focus away from the external impressions and creates peaceful and positive inner feelings is pratyahara. Detox from the media. Move your mind into a place of peace. Focus the inner eye, and the senses will follow. Exercise patience and practice.

- Dharana – Concentration: Today, we call this mindfulness. Here are a few suggestions from a 2015 article in BeYogi.com, *Before You Meditate, Concentrate: The Yogic Practice of Dharana*, to help you learn to be mindful.

  1. Stop multitasking. Whatever you are doing, do it with everything you have. Fully immerse yourself in every aspect of each activity you are doing.

  2. Practice Trataka:
     Sit comfortably with the spine erect.
     Place an object such as a burning candle, flower, stone, etc. at eye level.

Stare at an object for a few minutes without blinking or moving around.

Close your eyes and visualize that object. When it is gone, open your eyes and stare at it again.

Close your eyes and recall its color, shape, texture, form.

- Dhyana – Meditation: Focus on an object until you feel as if you are that object.

- Samadhi – Self-realization: According to Jafree Ozwald at www.enlightenedbe-ings.com, there are eight steps to achieving this state.

1. Approach life as if everyone and everything was put here just to teach you. Believe it or not, everyone has something from which you can learn, so it's important to dig for those gems within each person you meet. Having this mindset causes you to value the people you cross paths with, and it causes you to appreciate the path.

2. Don't worry about how anyone thinks of you. We are all on our unique journey—respect where you are and the circumstances that brought you

there. Do the same for others as well. Remember that no one's journey is better than anyone else's.

3. Honor the infinite power behind your word and thoughts. You can make or break anyone's day with your words. Your words are reflections of your thoughts, so guard your thoughts and reject negative ones to stay mindful of your words.

4. Be Fully Awake To The Now. Being present means to not dwell on the past or worry about the future. Embrace each moment for what it is: all you ultimately have.

5. Trust Your Experience. If it isn't right, it isn't done. Trust in the greater good to make all things work together for eventual good.

6. Reveal and Heal Your Shadow Side. No one honestly thinks you're perfect, so stop wasting energy trying to act like you are. Be honest with yourself and others as you strive toward a better version of yourself.

7. Respond To People Consciously. Be fully present with each interaction you have. To love is to give attention. Be attentive.

8. Let Go, Love, and Laugh! Don't take yourself or anything or anyone so seriously. Find the beauty and humor in everything, and just enjoy the ride.

Since Patanjali created the Yoga Sutra, it became widely popular in India, with many teachers adapting their specific spin to the sutras, eventually spreading around the globe. In 1893, the Chicago Parliament of Religions invited a yoga teacher from India named Swami Vivekananda to enlighten their attendees. His speech was so novel and well received that the audience gave him a standing ovation. Yoga became an American pastime. Since that introduction, yoga has evolved in the United States to include several different types of disciplines, including some pretty weird stuff such as Goat Yoga (Goats wander around, climbing all over you, while you work out). There is also Naked Yoga (...Yep.) But the five most popular styles of yoga in the United States are Hatha, vinyasa, hot, restorative, and ashtanga.

Types of Modern Yoga

Hatha yoga - This includes any type of yoga that combines movement with breath. Hatha yoga is the perfect introduction to yoga for beginners.

Vinyasa yoga - People consider this to be the next level up from Hatha yoga. Its focus is a more dynamic flow of postures that marry each breath to a movement with a relatively rapid flow between poses.

Hot Yoga - This type of yoga turns the temperature up, literally. The studio can be as hot as 120 degrees with 40% humidity. The idea behind hot yoga is greater flexibility and detoxification through sweat. The teachers recommend that you drink lots of water and wear light, breathable clothing.

Restorative yoga - The concept behind restorative yoga is to reach a state of deep relaxation for the body. Instructors provide props such as blocks, ropes, balls, and cushions so that you are comfortable enough to hold the various asanas for five minutes or more.

Ashtanga yoga - This is an athletic style of yoga and appeals to many people who want to take yoga to a much more intense level. The entire session will physically and mentally challenge you, and it is not for the beginner.

Vagus Nerve Yoga

Dr. Arielle Schwartz is a licensed psychologist who encourages vagus nerve yoga. She lists seven yoga practices that will stimulate the vagus nerve in a December 2017 post on her website (https://drari-elleschwartz.com).

Breathwork. Pranayama yoga is a form of poses that coordinates movement with breath. To bring about a greater sense of relaxation, make sure the exhale's length exceeds the duration of your inhale.

Smile. Try relaxing your face during your practice, but curve the corners of your mouth up into a gentle smile. Smiling will lighten your mood and, according to Dr. Porges, engage your "social nervous system," the most evolved branch of the vagus nerve.

Wake up. Yoga is the best way to wake up in the morning gently. It is also a refreshing way to perk up when you feel sluggish in the afternoon. Below is a description of Sun Salutations, which incorporates most of these vagus nerve yoga strategies. It is a fantastic way to start each day.

Release your belly. When you relax the muscles of your abdomen, you're making a connection with your vagus nerve.

Practice conscious compassion. According to Dr. Schwartz, people who practice kindness experience an increased vagal tone with a more exceptional ability to switch back and forth between the SNS and ANS as needed. They have an increased sense of social connectedness and more positive emotions.

Yoga Nidra. Dr. Schwartz recommends that you "find a relaxing position lying on the floor, blanket, or yoga mat, and cultivate awareness of your body and breath. Make space for whatever you are feeling, including any areas of tension, heaviness, or constriction. Allow yourself to remain still for 30 minutes for a deeply relaxing and nourishing experience."

Sunrise Salutations

For every *inhale*, use your diaphragm to fill your chest, drawing breath through your nose, expanding your ribs as much as possible. Try to make each inhale last for five seconds.

For every *exhale*, gently, slowly use your diaphragm to push the breath out of your lungs through your nose, making an ocean-like roar at the back of your closed mouth. One way to learn this sound is to exhale with your mouth open as if you were trying to fog up a mirror. Now do that again, but with your mouth closed. Try to make each exhale last for eight seconds.

Relax your face and then slightly turn up your lips into a gentle smile. Stand up straight and reach tall into a mountain pose. Your elbows are bent with your hands at your chest, as in prayer. Practice breathing, as detailed above. *Inhale* for a count of five. *Exhale* for a count of eight. *Inhale. Exhale.*

Inhale deeply while raising your arms straight up over your head and pushing your pelvis forward, tightening your thighs. Continue inhaling as you open your heart by bending your spine backward as far as you safely can without overdoing it. Stretch your arms up and back.

Exhale as you bend forward at your waist into a forward fold with your knees only slightly bent. Point your tailbone up with your arms dangling down and your hands as close to your feet as possible. Your goal over time will be to have your hands flat on the floor next to your feet.

Inhale as you move your right foot back as far as you can into a lunge position. Press your heel down to lengthen your spine.

Hold the breath as you bring your left foot back to your right foot to form a plank position.

Exhale as you bend your elbows while lowering your entire body to the floor in a low push-up position.

Inhale as you push your upper body up into the cobra position with your arms straight and your head back while your lower body remains lying on the floor.

Exhale as you lift your tailbone, bend your knees, and push your arms back into the child's pose. Lay your upper body over your thighs with your arms stretched out on the floor in front of you. *Inhale. Exhale.*

While you are breathing in child's pose, think of someone going through a difficult time right now. Empathize with them by trying to imagine how they must specifically feel about some aspect of their challenge. Concentrate on how this gives rise to feelings of compassion within you. Now think of a similar problem you've been through and transfer those feelings of kindness to yourself. If child's pose is too painful for your knees to stay here long, do this exercise of compassion in mountain pose.

Inhale, pushing your legs to a tabletop position; hands underneath your shoulders; knees underneath your hips. Continue inhaling as you let your belly sag down, look up, and flex your spine into the cow position.

Exhale as you curve your spine up, lower your head with your gaze at your belly button, and pull your belly up toward your spine in the cat position.

Inhale as you return to the tabletop position. Continue inhaling as you let your belly sag down, look up, and flex your spine in the cow position.

Exhale as you tuck your toes under, lift your tailbone upwards and straighten your legs into down dog position.

Inhale as you move your right foot forward between your hands into a lunge position. Press your heel back to lengthen your spine.

Exhale, bringing your left foot forward beside your right foot, and your waist bent into forward fold again.

Inhale while raising your arms high up over your head and pushing your pelvis forward, tightening your thighs. Continue inhaling as you open your heart by bending your spine backward as far as you safely can without overdoing it. Stretch your arms up and back, just as you did before.

Exhale into another mountain pose with your hands at your chest, as in prayer.

Repeat the entire sequence two more times

CHAPTER 17

Heart Rate Variability and Vagal Nerve Stimulation

The best way to measure the vagus nerve function is by heart rate variability (HRV). This measurement is very complex and includes the interaction of multiple systems. To simplify things, it shows how well balanced your sympathetic and parasympathetic nervous systems are. If you have made poor living choices, or your stress and anxiety levels are too high, your sympathetic nervous system will remain on overdrive. This situation will cause your resting heart rate to be too high, and your HRV will be too low. A large quantity of research published over the past 50 years correlates HRV to:

- Risk and progression of chronic diseases such as diabetes, cardiovascular disease, respiratory diseases, gastrointestinal diseases, autoimmune conditions, etc.

- Biological aging and health
- Physical performance (Elite endurance and team sports heavily use HRV to guide training and recovery)
- Injury prevention
- Guided rehabilitation
- Mental health, mood, depression, anxiety, PTSD
- Mental cognition
- Morbidity and mortality

HRV can be measured precisely in a laboratory, or you can measure it yourself. If you use the right tools, you can achieve a fairly decent degree of accuracy. Heart rate variability biofeedback (HRVB) has been gaining popularity because it allows you to see your progress. Using an app on your smartphone, you can see and adjust the differences you are making in strengthening your vagal tone.

One HRVB device recommended by Dr. Navaz Habib, author of Activate Your Vagus Nerve, is the Inner Balance tool from HeartMath. The Inner Balance tool can be used with your smartphone to track your HRV over time using a monitor that attaches to your earlobe and plugs into your phone. The HRV is calculated and displayed as a graph. The app then leads you through a meditative breathing exercise that, when followed to the end of the practice, should lead you into a state of coherence. Coherence is the synchronization of the HRV, respiration, and blood pressure into a rhythmic pattern. When you reach coherence, the heart, mind, and emotions are in a perfect state of oneness, which reduces stress. Coherence shifts the body toward increased parasympathetic activity, which translates to a firmer vagal tone.

According to the HeartMath website, the Inner Balance is recommended by thousands of health professionals and used by many hospitals, corporations, schools, and humanitarian organizations. Over 26 years of research has produced more than 300 independent peer-reviewed studies. Research conducted with 11,903 people have shown improvements in mental & emotional well-being in just 6-9 weeks using HeartMath training and technology:

24% improvement in the ability to focus

30% improvement in sleep

38% improvement in calmness

46% drop in anxiety

48% drop in fatigue

56% drop in depression

So, what does this data have to do with VNS? Vagal nerve stimulation has had mixed degrees of success in treating epilepsy and depression. Some people have responded quite well to it, while others didn't respond at all. There hasn't been a tool for predicting whether a patient would be significantly helped by VNS or not helped. But a recent study has illuminated some hope on this perplexing problem. It was explained in a 2018 Scientific Reports, *Preoperative Heart Rate Variability as Predictors of Vagus Nerve Stimulation Outcome in Patients with Drug-resistant Epilepsy* by Hong-Yun Liu et al. In this study, they looked at the HRV of drug-resistant epilepsy patients before receiving VNS surgery. They found that the lower the HRV was in the patient, the less likely they would be to respond to the VNS. This finding is significant because it can help doctors know whether to prescribe VNS to a patient.

A later study reported in October 2018 of Epilepsia cited the above investigation and furthered the research. This study by Kenneth A. Myers, et al. was titled *Heart rate variability measurement in epilepsy: How can we move from research to clinical practice?* Their objective was to evaluate the literature surrounding HRV in people with epilepsy. They made recommendations as to how to do future research to improve integration into clinical practice. The key points they gleaned from their evaluation were:

- HRV studies suggest that sympathetic over-activity occurs in most forms of epilepsy
- A dysfunctional autonomic system appears to be most severe in those with temporal lobe epilepsy and drug-resistant epilepsy.
- Doctors can use HRV to predict response to VNS.
- The lack of consistently used protocol has limited heart rate variability research in epilepsy.
- To successfully use

- HRV measurements in clinical practice, Researchers need to create a standardized evaluation protocol.

A 2017 study was recorded in the Annals of Indian Academy of Neurology by Karthi Balasubramanian, K Harikumar, Nithin Nagaraj, and Sandipan Pati. It was titled *Vagus Nerve Stimulation Modulates Complexity of Heart Rate Variability Differently during Sleep and Wakefulness*. This study demonstrated that the VNS increased the complexity of HRV during sleep and decreased it during wakefulness. They also found an increase in parasympathetic tone is associated with the increased complexity of HRV even in the presence of reduced heart rate.

These studies all involved the implanted VNS device, which, because of its semi-permanent nature and intrusive complications, may not appeal or even be available to the majority of the population. A 2016 study by Tiffany Truong and Rustin Berlow was published in the U.S. Psychiatric and Mental Health Congress Conference and Exhibition. This investigation tested the effects of transcutaneous vagal nerve stimulation (nVNS) on HRV. The participants received twenty minutes of auricular branch nVNS. Only during the last five minutes did they experience a significant increase in HRV.

HeartMath, described above, has a particular protocol for measuring and interpreting HRV. According to HeartMath, the most common way to measure HRV is to quantify the variations. However, this calculation does not reflect the emotional states of the individual and, therefore, doesn't give a complete picture. A more accurate measure is to focus on the amplitude of the wave and rhythm pattern.

The amplitude is naturally related to one's age. The younger you are, the higher your HRV. If you have a lower than average HRV for your age, this is indicative of future health problems and low resilience to stress. The lowering of the HRV score does not go down suddenly unless someone is subjected to extreme trauma or develops a clinical disorder like diabetes. Instead, over months and years, because of stress and aging, the HRV score may decrease.

Also, the score will vary depending on the time of day and mood. Specialists recommend that you take your HRV reading at the same time to maintain consistency. This recommendation is because HRV follows a circadian rhythm. Your HRV peaks at night between 10 pm and 2 am. This peak is when the body is most relaxed because nighttime is when your body makes much of its essential recovery and repair. Your HRV is the lowest between 9 am and noon. This interval is probably your most active time of day, so it's not surprising that your body has turned off the rest and digest response. Not only does your average value of HRV get lower as you age, but your night-day variation also reduces as you get older. You will also have a lower average HRV if you are depressed or have low-grade inflammation.

Surprisingly though, HRV is independent of heart rate. You can have a high heart rate and still have a good HRV. Conversely, you can have a low heart rate and have a low HRV, never reaching coherence. Your heart rate increases as you breathe in, and it goes down as you breathe out.

Furthermore, as blood pressure increases, heart rate goes down. And as blood pressure decreases, heart rate goes up. This correlation is caused by the baroreflex, which is a complicated feedback loop to ensure your brain always receives an adequate amount of blood. However, a rising heart rate does not cause your blood pressure to increase at the same rate. While your heart beats more times a minute, healthy blood vessels get larger to allow more blood to flow smoothly. When you are active, your heart rate goes up, so more blood can reach your working muscles. It may safely be possible for your heart rate to double. At the same time, your blood pressure may respond by only increasing a little bit. Your heart rate and blood pressure are intricately related. Your vagus nerve is continuously monitoring and balancing your heart rate and blood pressure. An isolated increase in blood pressure can indeed drop the heart rate a little. In some situations, both heart rate and blood pressure can decrease at the same time. Other times, both heart rate and blood pressure rise together, such as when you exercise or get angry.

It is possible to get a baseline reading that reflects your response to stress by forming a mental image of a stressful situation while recording your HRV. Compare that to an optimal baseline reading by breathing six breaths per minute to induce coherence. Another baseline reading can be taken for ten minutes when you are sitting quietly and breathing normally to see your typical resting HRV.

The Promise of Heart Rate Variability Biofeedback: Evidence-Based Applications by Richard Gevirtz is a study in a 2013 issue of ResearchGate. It outlines numerous studies that have found significant results in the use of HRVB for multiple disorders. He divided these benefits into three categories: restoring balance, central effects by way of the vagal afferent nerve, and the cholinergic anti-inflammatory system.

For restoring balance, Gevirtz lists asthma and chronic obstructive pulmonary disorder first for receiving powerful intervention by HRVB. Participants in the studies reported fewer symptoms and better lung function. Functional gastrointestinal disorders are also listed, which include esophageal pain and irritable bowel syndrome. He suggests that this application may hold the most promise for HRVB. Fibromyalgia is also listed, but the intervention consists of integrating other therapies as well, such as exercise, acceptance and commitment therapy, cognitive-behavioral therapy, and sleep hygiene. Paired with HRVB, these treatments have met with some success. Cardiac rehabilitation increasingly uses the balancing of the sympathetic with the parasympathetic nervous systems using HRVB as an exciting way to impact the heart muscle. When you use HRVB, you can strengthen the baroreflex to reduce hypertension. Sufferers of chronic muscle pain may also find hope in HRVB. Adding this to traditional back exercises and trigger point release produced some pain management. A final application for maintaining homeostasis through the use of HRVB is in obstetrics. The use of HRVB for conditions such as pregnancy-induced hypertension and preterm labor reduced symptoms and extended gestation by almost two weeks. This additional time allowed the birth of heavier, healthier babies due to increased developmental time.

Researchers recognized the use of HRVB for central effects by way of the vagal afferent nerve because of the positive findings of VNS on epilepsy and depression. The reasoning is that if electrical stimulation can reverse these diseases through deep brain stimulation, the use of slow breathing can stimulate vagal afferent nerves below the diaphragm. Regardless of how it works, users of HRVB report improvements in depression, anxiety, and sleep. These disorders and treatments involve cognition, mindfulness, and self-efficacy. As we will soon discover in the following chapter about yoga, brain scan studies show physical changes over time due to the deep breathing discipline associated with yoga and meditation.

At the time of Gevirtz's publication, researchers hadn't thoroughly looked into the benefits of HRVB on the anti-inflammatory system. However, there had been some very positive results showing a reduction in cytokine symptoms. This discovery could lead to applications such as treatment for autoimmune disorders and poor healing.

Gevirtz also mentions briefly in his study the effects of HRVB in optimal sport performance by way of the central effects of the vagal afferent nerve. There are so many studies in this area that it warrants a category of its own. A quick scan of the literature reveals HRVB to be effective in the researched performance of athletes in swimming, speed skating, archery, basketball, baseball, target shooting, golf, combat sports, gymnastics, tennis, etc. The commonality in the results of all these athletes, regardless of sport, seems to be heightened cognitive awareness, reduced stress and anxiety, quickened recovery time, and better gas exchange efficiency.

A 2012 study by Wells, Outhred, et al. titled *Matter Over Mind: A Randomized-Controlled Trial of Single-Session Biofeedback Training on Performance Anxiety and Heart Rate Variability in Musicians* in PubMed shows HRVB to be rather useful for the treatment and prevention of performance anxiety in musicians.

Another therapy that stimulates the vagus nerve and is gaining in popularity is PEMF. Doctors use Pulsed Electromagnetic Field therapy to improve the healing rate after injury, immune function, sleep, depression, bone healing and density, circulation, and overall body energy. It works by send-ing low voltage bursts of electricity through the skin and into muscles, bones, tendons, and even or-gans to boost the amount and the performance of your cell's mitochondria. The mitochondria are the power generators in your cells. They turn the food you eat into energy you can use. The more mito-chondria you have in each body cell and the better they are working, the more powerful you will feel. Research confirms that PEMF therapy stimulates the vagus nerve and increasing the HRV by using a device that stimulates pulsed magnetic field waves directly on the gut, head, and neck.

CHAPTER 18

How Yoga Improves Heart Rate

The following testimonies about yoga are from the 2016 documentary "My Dharma." Dharma is the eternal and inherent nature of reality. It is Truth. The practice of yoga transformed each person in the documentary. Besides all being able to do amazing poses with unbelievable flexibility and strength, they all shared a universal truth; a respect for life that they found through yoga.

Laruga Glaser found yoga in her search for spiritual truths. Yoga spoke to her, though, because it is experiential. You have to go through the process of performing the movements (asanas) to become internally aligned and to understand. Yoga, she says, changes you from the inside, making you want to be a good person and making you want to live more authentically. Laruga exuded a peace about her that she says she got from yoga.

Deepika Mehta from India fell 40ft. while rock climbing. She spent two years recovering in bed, and her doctors told her that she'd never walk again. Compelled to try yoga, Deepika not only re-learned how to walk but dances now too. She says the movement of yoga is her prayer; it is how she expresses devotion to God and self. She finds the daily practice of yoga makes her present to her patterns of the mind. This awareness, she feels, helps her to view other people as a mirror to parts of herself.

Liz Huntley from Canada and Roland Jensch from Germany practice yoga together. Yoga means union, Liz says. It is an individual practice, but doing it together forms relationships. They build off each other's strengths. Roland was successful at meditation. His daily practice encouraged Liz to stick with it, even though it was challenging for her.

Aline Fernandes from Brazil says that yoga lets you know who you are, which helps you relate better to others and nature.

Jessica Olie from Dubai says that it isn't about being better or more flexible than someone else in the class. The practice is about being better than you were yesterday.

Kino MacGregor literally radiates joy. She is from the United States and began taking yoga classes because she was depressed. During the first class, the teacher hummed a loud "Ohmmm," and the students joined. The resonance of the vibration spoke to her, and her soul answered back, "Yes." She has since moved to India and has devoted her life to living and teaching yoga. She says the asanas are vehicles toward a more profound knowing of oneself and a more in-depth knowing of God. She teaches that you recognize who you are when tested by approaching points of difficulty within yourself. "We don't truly know if we're peaceful people until we reach that moment of difficulty, to understand what it means to be strong on a spiritual level. Once you experience that inner knowing, you have more patience with yourself and ultimately with the whole world." Yoga, she says, is the path to knowing God and yourself. The beautiful acts of surrender help you realize that you won't find worth in achievement but your soul's quality.

Radha Rajani from Italy practices a more meditative form of yoga involving chanting and sound.
Through meditation, she says that we lose fear,
darkness, anger, and, most of all, ignorance. Then
we can meet and see ourselves as we are and see
everything as it is.

Hayley Cutler from Dubai practices Kundalini
yoga. This type of yoga has similar movements as
hatha yoga and incorporates mantras, meditation,
and dance. Hayley says that since beginning her
practice, it has been like coming home to oneself.
You remember who you indeed are.

Meghan Currie from Canada says it's like making
love to life, to nature, to all aspects of life that are
so precious and beautiful. After years of practice,
she went from following regimented sequences to a
more spontaneous flow, allowing her body to go
places before her mind knew what would be happening. The series unfolds now, and often she
doesn't even know what she did. "If we can trust
enough to say 'Ok, maybe I will mess up. Maybe I
won't know what to do, but let's just see, and who
cares if I don't know what to do.' Then we start to
be a little more pliable. We begin to give back the

trust to ourselves. After all, we always calculate every moment because we're afraid of messing up. But if we can give up this fear of making a mistake, we give the trust back to ourselves, and then we can really let ourselves unfold."

All of these people have found truths in doing yoga that they have been able to translate to other aspects of their lives. They have learned to trust themselves in any situation. They have learned to calm down through breathing. They have learned to respect life in all its forms. Their gentle practice has taught them patience, which translates into a peace that permeates all of their being. How does yoga do this? What generations of yogis have known, science is beginning to understand. The following doctors and scientists were interviewed in the 2016 documentary, The Science of Yoga. They take the previous anecdotes and back them up with data.

Michael de Manincor, a psychologist and Director of the Yoga Institute, reported his research findings. His study compared groups of people who suffer from depression. The group that did yoga, along with their usual medication, had a 33% reduction in anxiety after just doing yoga for twelve minutes a day.

Sat Bir Khalsa, Associate Professor of Medicine at Harvard Medical School reports in this same documentary that brain scan images show changes in brain activity during meditation. Over time, this activity will change the brain structure. Also, he reports that neurotransmitters are produced, and positive gene activity is enhanced. He recorded changes on the cellular and molecular level. He says four parts to yoga cause it to affect heart rate— first, the asanas and the pranayamas, the postures and the breathing. The discipline of doing these physical exercises and controlled breathing strengthens the HRV. Second, the self-regulation teaches resilience to stress, a mind over matter, if you will. Third, mind/body awareness increases mindfulness and lowers anxiety. Finally, if you achieve mastery over your fears, you will reach deeper states of transcendence. These moments may be brief, but they are enough to enhance life's meaning and push you farther into your discipline.

Dr. Mithu Storoni says that breathing, combined with the mind control necessary to do the asanas, is how yoga improves your health. "Breath is the most powerful tool that everyone has within their reach to bring their stress response under control." The most direct way, she says, is to take fewer breaths within an amount of time.

Dr. Bruce Lipton, a cell biologist who teaches epigenetics, says that the mind ultimately controls the body. He says that only 1% of illness is related to genes; 90% of disease is due to stress.

Laura Plumb, a natural medicine practitioner, says that yoga is excellent for improving health and healing. That is why many people get started on yoga's path. Still, yoga is so much more than that. Yoga is about the truth of knowing who you are, which is something that science may never be able to catch up.

The inner calm, the breathing discipline, and meditation all coincide with lower heart rate, reduce the stress response, lower blood pressure, and lighten the mood.

CHAPTER 19

How Exercise and Various Mind-Body Therapies Strengthen the Vagal Tone

If you've ever committed to an exercise program, you know from experience that the more you work at it, the better you become. Perhaps a recent physical exam at the doctor's office opens your eyes to the toll that time has on your body. You're almost 40, and your muscle tone is non-existent, both your belly and your chins have rolls, your blood pressure and resting heart rate are too high. At the same time, your HRV is too low, you haven't had any energy lately, nothing excites you, your brain feels foggy, and you can't even go upstairs without getting out of breath. You feel compelled to lose weight, get more fit, look better, and, most of all, feel better physically, mentally, and emotionally. So, with your doctor's approval, you decide to start a running program. Running is, after all, one of the most efficient ways to get fit and between work and the kids' busy schedules, you don't have a lot of time to spend on this new endeavor. You do some research and find Couch to 5K. It's a great program for beginning runners. Just as it says, it literally walks you through the training necessary to go from being a couch lounger to running your first 5k race.

You look over the plan, and you know you can do this; you used to run in high school, no problem. You buy the new shoes, the black spandex, the breathable tank. You haven't even started yet, and you already look better. You download some tunes that motivate you and get a pair of Bluetooth ear-buds. How can anything go wrong?

On your first attempt, everything goes wrong, and you can't even go a quarter of a mile without having to stop and rest. Your heart is violently pounding in your chest, and your lungs feel like they're on fire. How did you get this far out of shape? You plow forward, walking and running some, but it isn't anything like what you expected from yourself. Halfway out, you begin to have a mild anxiety attack at your turnaround point because you aren't sure if you can even make it back. Still, you hope no one drives by who knows you because this is just embarrassing. You feel nauseated and discouraged; maybe you even think that running just isn't for you. That night you can barely move. But for some reason, you find yourself out there again the next day, feeling equally discouraged. Plus, now your muscles ache from the previous day. This workout is even worse.

Nevertheless, you're determined to do this, so you get back out there, day after day, week after week. And you slowly begin to see results. That quarter of a mile turns into half a mile. That 14 minute per mile pace turns into a 13 minute per mile pace. Your jeans aren't as tight, you're sleeping better at night, and your self-confidence is getting just a bit of a boost. These positive outcomes turn into a feedback loop. You find yourself wanting to work even harder to get even better results. So, you pump up the volume. You find songs that have a higher beat per minute and shoes that are lighter and more flexible. Your mileage is going up, and your times are going down. Eventually, you can run three miles consistently without stopping at all.

As you finish your first race, you look back over the past year, and you almost want to laugh at yourself for those first workouts that seemed like torture. But you don't laugh at yourself. On the contrary, you're quite proud of yourself. You set a goal, pushed through the pain, didn't give up, and reached the finish line. You physically look better than you have in years and, even though you're still huffing and puffing from the race, you also feel better than you have in years. And your recovery time is nothing like it was a year ago. In fact, you plan to do some yard work when you get home from the race. Then, you plan to sign up for the next race!

Over the past year, some pretty amazing changes occurred mentally and physically. That first run you did was so painful because you actually were damaging and tearing your leg muscles. They were sore the next day because they were injured and trying to heal. When they did recover, though, they were a tiny bit stronger and more substantial than they previously were. Your lungs burned because you were breathing through your mouth, and your brain thought your lungs were losing too much carbon dioxide. In response, your lungs produced goblet cells to produce mucus, which slowed your breathing and constricted your blood vessels. This vasoconstriction and excess mucus made catching your breath more difficult, resulting in that painful burning sensation. As time went by, you learned how to breathe through your nose more and control your breathing. Breathing through your nose reassured your brain that all was well, and it relaxed, allowing you to develop a rhythm to your inhalations. Your heart was pounding because it's a muscle, and just like your leg muscles, the exertion made tiny tears throughout it. Just like your leg muscles, as you recovered, your heart was a little bit bigger and more powerful than before.

Even your brain changed because of running. By increasing your aerobic fitness, you also increased your neurotransmitters like serotonin and norepinephrine, causing your nervous system to generate new neurons. The stress your body experienced through running taught your brain that it could cope with discomfort. Oddly enough, this translated to other parts of your life as well. You found that little things such as traffic annoyances didn't bother you as much because your stress regulation response was more robust. You kicked your metabolism into a higher gear, and you found you could eat more, yet weigh less. But even your diet changed. Heavily processed foods, sugary desserts, bad fats; these meals made you feel sluggish and affected your ability to run, so you inherently avoided them. Eating healthier, in turn, made you more energetic and leaner. Another feedback loop: the better you ate, the better you felt; the better you felt, the better you ate.

At your next physical exam, the doctor was stunned by your metamorphosis. Your weight was down, your blood pressure was down, and your resting heart rate was down. Conversely, your HRV was up, your muscle tone was up, your mood was up, and your mental sharpness was more focused. What did you do? "I ran."

How does all this relate to your vagus nerve? If you've been following along in this book, I'll bet you can figure it out. What controls everything you just experienced while learning to run? What controls your heart rate, breathing, blood pressure, mood, anxiety, stress response, and even mental clarity? Yep. The vagus nerve.

In the July 10, 2018 Frontiers in Neuroscience, *Vagal Tank Theory: The Three Rs of Cardiac Vagal Control Functioning – Resting, Reactivity, and Recovery* by Sylvain Laborde, Emma Mosley, and Alina Mertgen, a new theory is introduced involving the vagus nerve. It builds on Dr. Steven Porges's Polyvagal Theory and the neurovisceral integration model proposed by Smith, R.and Thayer, J. F, and refined in 2017. This model suggests that emotional intelligence can predict the amount of control the vagus nerve has on heart rate (CVC-cardiac vagal control) and vice versa.

The Vagal Tank Theory uses a tank as a metaphor to explain how the CVC works. It involves three stages in the stress cycle: resting, reactivity, and recovery. The test consists of getting the resting HRV as a baseline, during a stressor (reactivity), and after the episode has passed (recovery) to compare with the initial baseline reading. An illustration shows the resting HRV as a ⅔ full tank. The reactivity stage shows a container that is either filled higher or lower, depending on how stressful the episode is. The amount of stress to which the individual is exposed determines the sympathetic versus parasympathetic response during the reativity phase. If the pressure is minimal, the vagal response will be higher in healthy subjects. If the provocation is high, the sympathetic response will be higher, and the vagal response will decrease. Therefore, recovery will also be affected. In the recovery tank illustration, depending on the individual's vagal tone, they will have a lower HRV, the same HRV, or a higher HRV. The researchers were able to conclude that cardiac vagal control has an overreaching influence on several vital self-regulatory aspects of behavior.

Another publication *applied the Tank Theory to exercise. Commentary: Vagal Tank Theory: The Three Rs of Cardiac Vagal Control Functioning – Resting, Reactivity, and Recovery*, by Hottenrotts et al. in ResearchGate. They expressed similar findings, but the illustrated tanks had two compartments symbolizing a lying down position when HRV is measured and a standing position when HRV is measured. The suggestion that reaction is the same whether the stressor is physical (exercise) or psychological (social, mental, etc.) implies that the results can translate across boundaries. In other words, a physically resilient person also has a more significant potential to be psychologically resistant to stress.

A study by Matos, Felipe & Vido, Amanda & Garcia, William & Lopes, Wendell Arthur & Pereira, Antonio in 2020 called *A Neurovisceral Integrative Study on Cognition, Heart Rate Variability, and Fitness in the Elderly* in Frontiers in Aging Neuroscience confirmed the relationship between mental function and HRV and physical fitness, particularly between working memory, cardiorespiratory fitness, and dynamic balance.

Qi Fu and Benjamin D. Levine published *Exercise and the Autonomic Nervous System* in the Handbook of Clinical Neurology, Vol. 117 (3rd series) Autonomic Nervous System. They reinforced the widely known conclusion that a sedentary lifestyle is one of the most changeable risk factors for morbidity and mortality in humans. Physical activity or exercise training is necessary to maintain overall health and functional capacity. It plays a crucial role in preventing inflammatory diseases such as cardiovascular disease, sudden cardiac death, hypertension, type II diabetes, colon cancer, breast cancer, and obesity. Exercise improves function in patients with autonomic disorders, such as orthostatic intolerance, syncope, or POTS. Also, exercise training improves mental health, helps prevent depression, and promotes or maintains positive self-esteem. Adaptations involving the autonomic nervous system play a significant role in the protective and therapeutic effects of exercise training.

Exercise is one of the very best therapies to strengthen the vagal tone. And just like a muscle, the more you work at it, the stronger and healthier it will become. Humans were made to move and, no matter what your fitness level, the more you build motion into your day, the healthier you will be. The above article recommends moderate-intensity exercise for at least 30 minutes per day and at least five days per week for the vast majority of people. The important thing is to find a form of exercise that you will enjoy enough to keep coming back. It helps to find a friend to work out with, someone who will push you and hold you accountable.

Other forms of mind-body therapies to strengthen the vagal tone include singing, ear acupuncture, and aromatherapy. Inhaling essential oils known to be relaxing, such as lavender or bergamot, increase HRV. If you don't have either of those, breathing in any scent that you enjoy can have beneficial effects. Previously mentioned activities to stimulate vagal tone are maintaining strong social relationships, eating a healthy diet, sleeping restfully on your side, and submerging yourself in cold water. Several more suggestions are in Chapter 8. The important thing is that you work at it. Your vagal tone is naturally going to decrease as you age, so it's up to you to maintain your HRV.

CHAPTER 20

Vagus Nerve- The Brain Modulator

Marina* was 28 when her life changed forever. And it's funny because she thought it had already changed forever. Nine years ago, Marina, a bright-eyed, naive college freshman, planned to change the world. But she was unthinkably betrayed by someone she thought could be trusted. A "friend" had asked her out on a date, slipped her a date rape pill, had his way, claimed she'd asked for it, and left her like trash. Yes, Marina had been drinking, and no, she didn't usually drink. Yes, Marina was very attracted to him. Still, no, she'd never been intimate before and didn't plan to be that night. Yes, her outfit was a bit revealing, but no... No!

Still, Marina didn't know what to believe, and she was too embarrassed to confront him. He was treating her like dirt now, and, for the first time in her young life, she felt like dirt. Then she found out she was pregnant. Shame and fear plagued her. Her parents were very conservative. How would they react? Should she just quietly have an abortion? Her upbringing made that impossible. Should she run away? How could she and the baby survive with no money, no education, no health care? She knew she had to go home and face her parents.

It wasn't easy. And at first, Marina's parents were upset. They believed her, but Marina could see their disappointment on their faces. Eventually, though, Marina's parents found the joy in knowing they were going to be grandparents. They had adopted Marina, who was their only child when she was just an infant. They had always wanted a big family. Despite the circumstances, they were getting excited about having another baby around the house. They had never had a lot of money, and they knew it would be challenging for them, but they weren't going to let Marina lose out on life. They were going to circle the wagons and make a happy home.

Once she had her parents' blessing and support, Marina returned to her old, happy, albeit pregnant, self. She had always been determined to make the most out of every situation, and this situation was no different. She'd go to the community college to get the classes she wanted. She'd come out on top, she knew it. She had always been a genuine health nut, but now she took it to the extreme. She exercised daily, ate a whole foods diet, got to bed early every night, read all the books about pregnancy, and even started yoga and meditation.

When she finally had the baby, Marina and her parents fell in love with the little infant boy. He had her dimples and curly dark hair. They named him Jeremiah, after the weeping prophet, because his start was so riddled with sorrow. But he never felt unwanted a day in his life even though they never kept his origins a secret.

Marina went on to get her degree in education and landed a teaching position at the local elementary school. As Jeremiah got older, he eventually attended her school. They spent their summers at the community pool, and they had friends over all the time. They even had a silly dog named Spot to complete the family.

So when Marina's life changed forever again, she was floored. She was actually at the pool one sunny afternoon in June when an exceptionally amiable stranger approached her and took the lounger next to hers. Jeremiah was on the other side of the pool playing with friends, and Marina was enjoying some rare alone time. The friendly stranger then called her Maria*. Marina had met many parents over the years as a teacher, and she assumed that it must be a parent who hadn't gotten her name right. But then the friendly stranger asked how her shift at the convenience store was last night. Marina was a bit taken aback. Why would this stranger think she was working at a convenience store last night? This misunderstanding was weird. She tried not to embarrass the woman but let her know that she must have her mixed up with someone else...

That was how Marina found out that her birth mother had actually had identical twins. Due to financial and emotional reasons, however, she chose to give one up in a closed adoption. Neither Marina nor Maria had known that they were part of a package deal. The friendly stranger got the twins reunited, and both their lives began a new trajectory.

At first, it was fun to compare all the quirky similarities; Maria also had a dog named Spot. But the differences between them were more startling than the similarities. Maria was a bit overweight; she smoked, she drank too much, her only social life involved the few friends who worked at the convenience store with her. Maria never exercised, and she struggled with diabetes, negativity, and depression. Maria didn't do well in school, but nothing particularly traumatic had ever happened to her other than that her mother had died of cancer a few years before. Although her mother had to work, sometimes two jobs, throughout Maria's childhood, she was close to her mother. Her death left Maria lonely and now, with many questions unanswered. She was grateful to have a sister now but was puzzled by their differences.

What would cause two people with identical genetics, to be so different? Of course, one's environment plays an immense role in how people turn out, but it isn't the answer to all of the differences. If anyone had had a traumatic event in her life, it was Marina.

It's impossible to know for sure why Maria and Marina were so different. Still, two words could explain many of the differences: epigenetics and resilience.

Epigenetics

Epigenetics is a relatively new science that is taking the research world by storm. It has been thought for years that our genes determine everything there is about who we are, how we look, and why we do what we do. And if it couldn't be determined by genetics, then it must be answered by our environment. But another factor is shedding some light on why we are who we are. Epigenetics is the study of how some genes are turned on, or expressed, and how others are turned off. These switches may have occurred because of choices or experiences our parents or even grandparents had.

A study describes this theory in the March 14, 2016 publication of The Conversation called *Epigenetics: Can stress really change your genes?* The grandchildren of the survivors of the 1944 Dutch famine were born underweight, even though their mothers had plenty of food while pregnant with them. The malnutrition suffered by their grandparents was expressed in them. We realize a greater understanding of how genes are expressed. We are finding that just because you are genetically inclined to have a disease doesn't mean you will have it. Your lifestyle choices may have more to say about that than your genes.

Sanders, Teresa & Weiss, Joseph et al. in 2019 published *Cognition-EnDespiteus Nerve Stimulation Alters the Epigenetic Landscape* in The Journal of Neuroscience. Their study provides critical insights into VNS-induced epigenetic alterations in pathways important for enhanced cognition. In other words, VNS can change which genes are activated to enhance memory and learning and affect behavior. Other studies have found that increased sympathetic nervous system activity (stress) turns on genes related to breast cancer and other cancers.

Interestingly, most of the factors influencing your genetic inheritance's expression also affect your vagal tone—diet, lifestyle, exercise, sleep habits, environmental factors, stress, and social relationships. As this study evolves, the vagus nerve may well play a significant part, the brain's modulator, by way of genetic expression.

Resilience

What makes one person look adversity in the face and rise above it while another person shrinks into a puddle of insecurity or self-pity? The dictionary defines resilience as the capacity to recover quickly from difficulties. When you imagine what you hope people will say about you at your funeral, one thing stands out: resilience. The most touching memorial services usually involve anecdotes of how the deceased never let things get him down. "She had a great attitude all the way until the end." "He was a fighter." "She had it rough growing up, but you'd never know it." "Despite his pain, he was always more concerned about other people."

Resiliency is the thing we seem to prize most. We root for the underdog. We laugh with the comedian who can poke fun at his life's hard knocks. We celebrate the unlikely team that pushes ahead to win. For some reason, we're hard-wired to respect success when it comes against all the odds. If you do a

TEDTalk search on resilience, there are many excellent selections available. Here are just a few.

Raphael Rose, a clinical psychologist who researches for NASA, says that facing our stress is an integral component of being more resilient. In his TEDxManhattan talk, he describes the types of stress astronauts face on the ISS. Surprisingly, they aren't very different from the stresses we face on Earth: how the kids are doing in school, complicated relationships with co-workers, financial worries, etc. After working with astronauts, he gives several suggestions to develop resilience in your own life. First of all, he says to make slow and gradual changes that are incremental enough for you to commit. Once one small change becomes a habit, then move on to another positive change. Secondly, he says to be compassionate with yourself. If you fall back a step, be kind as you encourage yourself to try again. Finally, he suggests engaging in meaningful pursuits that will help relieve stress. Start a hobby that you enjoy. Do something, anything, that brings joy into your life to distract you from your challenges.

Charles Hunt gave a TEDxCharlotte talk titled, *What Trauma Taught Me About Resilience*. Charles learned about resilience at an early age where, growing up in the projects, he lost his mother and father. Charles went on to earn his bachelor's and master's degrees in business. He became very successful, but he never forgot his earliest classroom, trauma. His advice to anyone who wants to turn tragedy into triumph is to have the right perspective. You can overcome challenges because of the adversity, not despite it. The trick is to know when to ask for help and to find meaning in it. It's ok to admit that you were a victim but refuse to accept that you are a victim.

Dr. Sasha Shillcutt, MD, MS, FASE, gave a talk titled, *Resilience: The Art of Failing Forward*. She showed an iceberg illustration with the smaller, visible part representing what people think builds resilience. The more substantial, submerged part, though, is what she says builds resilience. She shared qualities that resilient people have. Resilient people accept that failure will happen, and they don't try to hide it when it does. They seek feed-back from others about their defeat, and they move forward despite it.

Finally, Lucy Hone has been researching resilience her entire adult life. Still, it wasn't until the tragic death of her twelve-year-old daughter in an auto-mobile collision that she came to understand the bare facts of resilience. She gave a TEDxChrist-church talk titled, *The Three Secrets of Resilient People*. First, resilient people accept that suffering is part of all human existence. In an age of extreme entitlement, it's essential to understand that you will suffer and that no one is exempt. Also, resilient people seek and find the good, even in the midst of their suffering. They cultivate gratitude. Finally, she encourages everyone to ask themselves a simple question that can transform anyone's life. Always be mindful enough in all your activities, thoughts, and conversations of "Is this helping or harming me?" If you can be objective enough to evaluate your daily choices and deliberately turn from self-destructive thoughts, words, and deeds, it can build resilience.

So what do epigenetics and resilience have to do with the vagus nerve? The Autonomic Nervous system is one of balance and homeostasis. We were designed to be healthy, active, and social. The vagus nerve is our regulator of harmony, and if we can relax and allow it to do its job, we'll find peace and well-being. The problems arise when stress takes the upper hand, though. When the sympathetic nervous system becomes dominant, physical, mental, and emotional health, all take a hit.

As in the cases of Marina and Maria, although they had the same genetics, their lifestyle choices and paths determined the expression of those genes. Marina was adopted into a supportive family who made healthy lifestyle choices about diet, exercise, and social engagement. Her internal strength turned life's challenges into growth. Maria had less support. She hadn't grown up making healthy lifestyle choices and didn't know better as an adult. Her internal vigor was compromised.

Call it what you will, but resilience, internal strength, and vigor can all be controlled by the vagus nerve. How we protect and cultivate that inner harmony can literally determine which genes will be expressed and which genes will be suppressed. We have learned in this book that a robust social network is crucial to feeling safe. In Chapter 14, fear was said to be the second most potent force we face. What's the strongest? Love. Our social networks equip us with the most dominant force in the universe. We have also learned that mindful breathing can hijack a panicked, nervous system to restore calm. We have learned that healthy lifestyle choices can give our nervous system the tools needed to thrive and stay regulated. And we have learned about therapies and applications that can provide an added boost when we need more help.

Our brains are beautiful, sophisticated, dynamic organs that are doing everything possible to ensure our safety, growth, and happiness. But to do that correctly and make the right decisions, they need to be getting the correct information. Most of us today are not being chased by a bear, but we allow the stressful details of life to make our brains think we are. Eighty percent of the vagus nerve's job is to bring decision altering information to the brain. We have the ability to make sure that information is correct so that we can enjoy a life of resilience.

*Names have been changed to protect the identities of individuals. In some cases, the stories of a few individuals with similar details have been merged into one account.

FREQUENTLY ASKED QUESTIONS

Why is there so much focus on the vagus nerve lately? Well, it has been of interest in Eastern medicine for eons. It is becoming of importance to Western medicine recently because there has been success in treating various illnesses and maladies through the manipulation of it. Western medicine has finally begun to move away from medication as a cure for everything. A more holistic approach is becoming accepted.

Is it possible to injure the vagus nerve? Yes! The vagus nerve, like any nerve, can most definitely be damaged. It can be impinged through spinal misalignment. It can be surgically cut (intentionally or unintentionally). Tumors or a hiatal hernia can put pressure on it. Toxins in the blood can also damage it.

Can the vagus nerve heal? It depends on the injury. If a cut or nick compromises the integrity of the structure, or if toxins in the blood have damaged it, then no, it is irreparable. If it is just pinched or compressed, then yes, once the pressure is relieved, it can return to its original vitality.

What is a poor vagal tone? An under- or overactive vagus nerve is said to have a poor vagal tone. Poor vagal tone means that it is, for a variety of reasons, not functioning correctly.

How do I know if I have a poor vagal tone? Almost any chronic disease can probably be traced back to the vagal nerve. If you have heart disease, diabetes, Alzheimer's, Crone's disease, arthritis, etc., your vagal tone should be considered. If you have simultaneous symptoms that don't seem to be related, yet can't be treated, you may need to work on your vagal tone.

For what is vagus nerve stimulation used? Currently, vagus nerve stimulation (VNS) is used to treat epilepsy and depression. It is also being studied for headaches and inflammatory diseases such as arthritis.

Who needs vagus nerve stimulation? Patients who don't respond to medications for epilepsy or depression are the typical individuals considered for

VNS. Children and pregnant women who don't want the drugs' side effects are also discussed.

How are mental illness and the vagus nerve related? Many mental illnesses are a result of prolonged anxiety. The vagus nerve, when properly maintained, is designed to alleviate stress.

Are there natural ways to stimulate the vagus nerve? Absolutely! The vagus nerve can be boosted naturally by daily movement and exercise, proper nutrition, positive social interaction, yoga, meditation, acupuncture, cold water, intermittent fasting, humming or singing, deep breathing, adequate sleep, and even laughter.

Why is yoga beneficial to the vagus nerve? Yoga coordinates movement with breath. It engages the diaphragm to activate deep belly inhalations while the actions are designed to open joints for healthy circulation. The mind is focused, in a meditative state, on control. These are all stimulators of the vagus nerve, which result in health and vigor.

Does diet affect the vagus nerve? Just like a factory can't function properly without regular in-coming shipments of all the necessary production parts, the body can't work well without the required chemicals. A diet rich in many different vegetables, fruits, grass-fed meat, healthy fats, and eggs can provide most of those necessary chemicals. Likewise, if a factory is bogged down by dirt, clutter, unfinished products, and lazy employees, the productivity will decrease. A diet full of sugar, processed grains, dyes, unhealthy fats, and preservatives will compromise the efficiency of the processes that are necessary to vitality. The vagus nerve functions best if it has all the required chemicals to perform its essential tasks.

How are gut health and the vagus nerve related?
Gut health is also a relatively new concept in Western medicine. It is the community of bacteria, fungi, and even viruses that live in the intestines. Healthy communities are made up of a diverse population of certain types of these organisms. In contrast, unhealthy communities have low diversity and some undesirable types. The vagus nerve carries information from the microorganisms to the brain and information from the brain to the microorganisms and other organs. If the community is healthy, the

communications result in overall positive health. If the community is unhealthy, the information results in overall adverse health.

CONCLUSION

Thank you for making it through to the end of *The Vagus Nerve*, let's hope it was informative and able to provide you with all the tools you need to achieve your goals whatever they may be.

The next step is to put the information you've gathered here to work for you. If you are suffering from poor health, please begin to make lifestyle changes that will improve your vagal tone. The least complicated and most beneficial changes will be simply to eat right and exercise. You've heard that all your life but may not know how that looks when you boil it down. There are various diets on the market, and they all seem to say that theirs is the best. So, which is the best? The very best nutritional program is the one that ultimately works for you. That being said, you won't find a single successful diet that promotes sugar, unhealthy fats, and highly processed foods. Start by getting rid of those three things, and you'll be amazed at how quickly your health will improve. If you search Dr. Edward

Dodge, you will find books and wellness newsletters packed with sound nutritional advice. He was practicing functional medicine decades before functional medicine even became a thing.

What exercise program is the best one? Again, the very best exercise is the one that ultimately works for you! Just move and find a way to enjoy it. If you enjoy it enough, you'll make a habit of it. Maybe you don't think you can enjoy exercise. Do you enjoy brushing your teeth? Probably not, but most people take the time to do it anyway. The same thing applies to working out. Commit to it and do it. Try to incorporate activities that build strength, make you breathe, opens your joints, and stretches your muscles. Yoga, done correctly, can include these things.

Beyond diet and exercise, the next most beneficial thing you can do for your vagal tone is to find positive, face-to-face social interaction. Put your phone down and find real people: join a club, go to church, take a class, volunteer, strike up a conversation in the break room. If you're into multitasking, find a friend to work out with, then get a green smoothie together afterward. Watch your conversation and try to keep it positive.

Then what? Have some fun: play and laugh and sing and cuddle a furry friend. Put deliberate joy into your life. Try new things: massage, acupuncture, meditation, cold showers, hot yoga.

But if you have epilepsy or your problems can't be resolved despite doing all of the above, consider vagus nerve stimulation. It may be precisely what you need to turn your life around.

Finally, if you found this book useful in any way, a review on Amazon is always appreciated!

CPSIA information can be obtained
at www.ICGtesting.com
Printed in the USA
BVHW091509170321
602801BV00010B/512